Talking about Treatment

OXFORD STUDIES IN SOCIOLINGUISTICS
Edward Finegan, *General Editor*

ENGLISH IN ITS SOCIAL CONTEXTS
Essays in Historical Sociolinguistics
Edited by Tim W. Machan and Charles T. Scott

COHERENCE IN PSYCHOTIC DISCOURSE
Branca Telles Ribeiro

SOCIOLINGUISTIC PERSPECTIVES ON REGISTER
Edited by Douglas Biber and Edward Finegan

GENDER AND CONVERSATIONAL INTERACTION
Edited by Deborah Tannen

THERAPEUTIC WAYS WITH WORDS
Kathleen Warden Ferrara

SOCIOLINGUISTIC PERSPECTIVES
Papers on Language in Society, 1959–1994
Charles Ferguson
Edited by Thom Huebner

THE LINGUISTIC INDIVIDUAL
Self-Expression in Language and Linguistics
Barbara Johnstone

THE DISCOURSE OF CLASSIFIED ADVERTISING
Exploring the Nature of Linguistic Simplicity
Paul Bruthiaux

QUEERLY PHRASED
Language, Gender, and Sexuality
Edited by Anna Livia and Kira Hall

CLAIMING POWER IN DOCTOR-PATIENT TALK
Nancy Ainsworth-Vaughn

KIDS TALK
Strategic Language Use in Later Childhood
Edited by Susan Hoyle and Carolyn Adger

TALKING ABOUT TREATMENT
Recommendations for Breast Cancer Adjuvant Therapy
Felicia D. Roberts

Talking about Treatment

Recommendations for Breast Cancer Adjuvant Therapy

FELICIA D. ROBERTS

New York Oxford
OXFORD UNIVERSITY PRESS
1999

Oxford University Press

Oxford New York

Athens Auckland Bangkok Bogotá Buenos Aires Calcutta
Cape Town Chennai Dar es Salaam Delhi Florence Hong Kong Istanbul
Karachi Kuala Lumpur Madrid Melbourne Mexico City Mumbai
Nairobi Paris São Paulo Singapore Taipei Tokyo Toronto Warsaw

with associated companies in
Berlin Ibadan

Published by Oxford University Press, Inc.
198 Madison Avenue, New York, New York 10016

Library of Congress Cataloging-in-Publication Data
Roberts, Felicia D.
Talking about treatment : recommendations for breast cancer adjuvant therapy / Felicia D. Roberts.
p. cm.
Includes bibliographical references and index.
ISBN 0-19-512191-0
1. Breast—Cancer—Adjuvant treatment. 2. Physician and patient.
3. Patient education. 4. Communication in medicine. I. Title.
RC280.B8R585 1998
616.99'44906—dc21 98-17829

1 3 5 7 9 8 6 4 2

Printed in the United States of America
on acid-free paper

For my parents

Series Foreword

Sociolinguistics is the study of language in use. With a special focus on the relationships between language and society, sociolinguistics addresses the forms and functions of variation across social groups and across the range of communicative situations in which speakers and writers deploy their verbal repertoires. In short, sociolinguistics examines discourse as it is constructed and co-constructed, shaped and reshaped, in the interactions of everyday life and as it reflects and creates the social and mental realities of life, as well sometimes of physical realities.

Some linguists examine the structure of sentences independent of who is speaking or writing and to whom, independent of what precedes and what follows in the discourse, and independent of the setting, topic, and purpose of the discourse. By contrast, sociolinguists and discourse analysts investigate linguistic expression embedded in its social and situational contexts. Among observers who are *not* professional linguists, interest likewise focuses on language in discourse—for it is discourse that mirrors the patterns of social structure and strategic enterprise that engage the attention of so many people.

Oxford Studies in Sociolinguistcs offers a platform for studies of language use in communities around the globe. The series invites synchronic or diachronic treatments of social dialects and registers, of oral, written, or signed discourse. It welcomes studies that are descriptive or theoretical, interpretive or analytical. While its volumes usually report original research, an occasional one synthesizes or interprets existing knowledge. The series aims for a style that is accessible beyond linguists to other humanists and social scientists, and some volumes may appeal to educated readers keenly interested in the language of human affairs—for example, the discourse of lawyers engaging clients and one another with specialist registers or, as in this volume, of oncologists and patients talking about suitable treatment. By providing a forum for innovative studies of language in use, Oxford Studies in Sociolinguistics aims to influence the agenda for linguistic research in the twenty-first century and to provide an array of provocative analyses to help launch that agenda.

In *Talking about Treatment*, Felicia D. Roberts thoroughly analyzes hours of talk between oncologists and patients after the patients have undergone surgery for breast cancer. At a time when health care providers increasingly recognize the pivotal therapeutic role of talk between physicians and patients, *Talking about Treatment* privileges the details of talk-in-interaction between physicians and patients, and it subjects a substantial sample of such talk to the tools of conversation analysis. *Talking about Treatment* reveals to physicians and patients alike the role of successful interaction in agreeing on treatments that are well understood by patients. In this important treatise Dr. Roberts has examined how patients and physicians co-construct "expertise." Her study aligns itself with other discourse studies that examine the dynamics of jointly and cooperatively constructing power and expertise. Taking a sophisticatedly naive view in her analyses, Dr. Roberts arrives at an understanding that can help bring about a more therapeutic balance of power and expertise in doctor-patient talk.

We are pleased to have *Talking about Treatment* as the latest contribution to Oxford Studies in Sociolinguistics.

Edward Finegan

Acknowledgments

I am indebted to many colleagues, teachers, family members and friends for making this book possible. Those named here and numerous others unnamed have contributed greatly to this project. I alone take responsibility for any shortcomings, but gladly share with them all of the good stuff.

First, a monumental "thank you" to Laura Siminoff who kindly shared her hard-earned data with me. Without her generosity and open mind, this work might never have been realized.

To my colleagues and the staff in the Department of Communication at Purdue University for their assistance as I worked on finishing this book, I extend thanks to them all.

Special acknowledgment goes to the faculty and staff of the University of Wisconsin-Madison, particularly those in the Department of English and the program for English Language and Linguistics. They trained me rigorously as a linguist and supported my development as a conversation analyst.

Cecilia Ford must take special credit for this project. She has read innumerable versions of this manuscript, yet never faltered in her enthusiasm for the research. Her skill as a conversation analyst and as a reader, along with her wisdom and kindness, made my job easier.

Polly Newcomb encouraged and supported my efforts as a health researcher and set the excellent example of her own rigorous scholarship. She graciously helped me find financial support for this project during its earliest stages, and in that regard I thank her, Pat Remington, and the Wisconsin Breast and Cervical Cancer Screening Project.

Virginia Gill and Tim Halkowski must also accept my heartfelt thanks. They have devoted much personal time to reading and critiquing my work and to thinking out loud with me. I shall always think of them with great respect and admiration for their own scholarship and for what they have shared with me.

Profound thanks to family and friends for their unending patience and support. Their love, respect, and sense of humor have kept me moving ahead, and that is what is at the core of this work.

And finally, to the unsung heroes of this kind of undertaking: the anonymous reviewers for Oxford University Press whose insightful and careful commentary helped to shape this book; to Elizabeth Ragsdale for her expert and patient technical assistance in preparing this manuscript for publication; and to the editors and production department at Oxford University Press for their flexibility and good humor—I appreciate all of your efforts and sincerely thank you for your help.

Contents

Talking about Treatment

1

Research Concerns and Review of Literature

How treatment recommendations are structured and delivered by doctors, and how they are received by patients, is a comparatively new area of study within the field of health communication. More specifically, very little research is available on medical recommendations as an accomplishment of talk-in-interaction. This study is intended to contribute in that regard; it is the first to present a qualitative analysis of the verbal interaction between oncologists and patients as they talk about treatment for breast cancer. As such, this book provides a foundation for further inquiry. We will look both at and around the treatment recommendation to account for the full range of activities that support and characterize this particular type of clinic visit. In this way, we get a glimpse at not only how patients and doctors come to an understanding about treatment options but also how, together, they structure the encounter as a legitimate occasion for expert advice-giving.

The medical visits to be investigated here are discussions between women who have undergone surgery for breast cancer and oncologists. The data are 22 audiotaped conversations (about 15 hours) in which the patient and doctor discuss, among other things, recommendations for adjuvant treatments, such as chemotherapy, radiation, and hormonal therapy. Most breast cancer patients are referred to oncologists by their primary care doctor or by their surgeon to discuss these adjuvant treatments in detail. The purpose of this book is to explore the artful management of these emotionally difficult and technically complex recommendation visits.

1.1 Research on Cancer Treatment Recommendations

Most research on breast cancer treatment recommendations has appeared in the medical literature within the past 10 years. The central concern of this work has been to discern whether or not there is an age bias in the treatment of cancer, and it appears that older women receive more conservative treatment than do younger women.[1] Other researchers have additionally tried to understand what contributes to these patterns of differential treatment. This work has relied on either vignette (Amir, 1987; Liberati et al., 1990) or retrospective approaches (Newcomb & Carbone, 1993). Importantly, Newcomb & Carbone (1993) reveal that both doctor recommendations and patient preferences affect selection of breast cancer treatments. From a methodological perspective, however, retrospection methodologies rely on the patient's memory of distant and emotionally troubling events to reconstruct what might have been advised during the clinic visit. Vignette studies (which present physicians with hypothetical patient profiles) tap physician beliefs about treatment, not necessarily their actual practice in a clinic setting. The gap between what a physician—or any other person—says they do, or might do, or would do can easily be different from what the person actually does. For this reason, it is important to inspect the actual talk that goes on between doctors and their patients if one is trying to explain or describe the medical dynamic.

Contemporaneous with the studies published in the medical literature, a pioneering series of quantitative investigations examined discussions between breast cancer patients and oncologists to better understand why some women follow treatment recommendations while others do not (Siminoff, 1987; Siminoff & Fetting, 1989, 1991; Siminoff, Fetting, & Abeloff, 1989). More recently, Ford, Fallowfield, and Lewis (1996) used a highly refined coding approach to investigate audiotaped "bad news" consultations (of various types) in oncology.

In the early study of breast cancer treatment recommendation visits (Siminoff, 1987) consultations were audiorecorded, then patient talk and doctor talk were coded for a predetermined list of topics, who initiated the topics, and the doctor's positive or negative framing of the prognosis. Post-clinic visit questionnaires were also administered. Of the 11 variables isolated for discriminating treatment acceptors from nonacceptors, the physician's recommendation was the strongest. Indeed 80% (n = 80) of

Siminoff's subjects chose the primary treatment option offered (Siminoff & Fetting, 1991). However, that finding, while instructive, leaves unanalyzed the complexity of the talk that surrounds and supports the recommendation. What is it in the talk that makes the recommendation compelling or, conversely, makes it unappealing? What happens when patients resist the recommendation?

Because the current study uses the audiotape data collected by Siminoff (1987), it is an excellent opportunity to fill in some of the details about oncologist-patient communication that the earlier quantitative analyses were not able to capture. For example, Siminoff et al. (1989) find that patients have an "extremely poor" understanding of the risks and benefits of treatment. Perhaps the equivocal nature of the discussion about risks and benefits (as discussed in detail in chapter 5 of this volume) is contributing to patient confusion. Without attention to the contributions of both patients and doctors in their full sequential context, this insight is easily missed. Such attention to qualitative detail allows us to flesh out more abstract analyses of medical interaction and breathe some life back into data that were, at the time of collection, lively and vibrant conversations.

In the only other study of doctor-patient talk in the context of cancer treatment recommendations, Fisher (1983) uses ethnographic methods supported by audiotaped records to study recommendations for treatment of dysplasia of the cervix (a precancerous condition). Drawing on the conceptual frameworks of speech act theory and the ethnography of speaking, Fisher relies on verbal interactions for her analysis and argues that information exchange, accomplished through *questioning* and *presentational* and *persuasional* strategies, shapes the decision-making process and the final treatment outcome (pp. 142–143). However, the analysis seems to be based more on assumptions about the doctor's attitude toward his patient than on an analysis of the talk itself: "I suspect that he [the physician] had already judged her [the patient] to be incompetent on grounds that are not displayed in the verbal communication between them. These assumptions structured the exchange of information that followed and had an impact on the treatment recommended" (p. 146). It is somewhat confusing to claim that information exchanged through a strategy such as questioning shapes a treatment recommendation when actually one is assuming that the physician's underlying biases shape the direction of the talk. Although I do not dispute that physician attitudes affect their interactions with patients (and probably that patient attitudes affect their interactions with doctors), I maintain Fisher's treatment of the data—the talk itself—is not convincing in that regard.

This study does not propose to answer the complicated array of questions about the sources of treatment bias. Rather, it deepens our understanding of how treatment recommendations are formulated, presented, and at times resisted in the moments of actual interactions. The current investigation begins with only one assumption, and that is that both patient and doctor contributions are consequential for the shape of the visit (and possibly for outcomes) and therefore analyzes the talk of both participants.

1.2 Analytic Approach and Research Questions

The current investigation contributes to earlier research on breast cancer treatment recommendations by taking an analytic stance that puts talk at the center of the analysis and provides access to that talk through detailed transcriptions of the audiotaped clinic visit. In this way, the reader has access to the conversation in nearly the same way that the analyst did at the time the analytic work was undertaken.

The approach here is to privilege the finely detailed, empirically verifiable aspects of talk-in-interaction. This is the theoretical and methodological foundation of conversation analysis (CA). Within this framework, sequential organization is a central concern (Psathas, 1995; Sacks, Schegloff, & Jefferson, 1974; Schegloff & Sacks, 1973; Zimmerman & Boden, 1991) and, given the constraint on analysis which calls for strict attention to adjacent utterances, context is understood as locally constructed.[2]

This approach differs from other discourse perspectives in that it treats context not as an external phenomenon shaping discourse but as something shaped through participant talk and action (see also Pomerantz & Fehr, 1997; Schegloff, 1992, 1997). As Drew and Heritage (1992) describe it, conversation analysis provides an "empirical analysis of the nature of context" (p. 17). Sociopolitical constructs are not viewed as driving the interaction, and analysts refrain from presupposing that any particular construct (e.g., power or gender) is shaping the talk. By attending to the sequential details of verbal and nonverbal interaction, it becomes apparent how the participants are creating a context through their local orientation to moments in the ongoing talk (Pomerantz & Fehr, 1997, pp. 66–70). In this way, it is possible to see what constructs or roles the participants make relevant (or not) and how they accomplish that "work" through interaction.

Indeed, as soon as I began working with the conversational data for this study I was struck by two things: (1) how much talk goes on before reaching the discussion of treatment options and (2) how the process of the visit, from beginning to end, conveys a feeling that doctors are trying to persuade patients to accept a particular adjuvant treatment, although they are unable to guarantee its curative power. Neither observation is necessarily startling, though each requires investigation.[3]

Treatments for breast cancer are standardized by the National Cancer Institute and updated as new findings become available. Oncologists can simply offer the currently standard treatment for the patient's particular case and, if the risks and benefits are acceptable to her, proceed to prescribe a regimen. Conceivably, then, doctors could prescribe adjuvant treatments without engaging in lengthy discussions with patients. Yet the oncologists in this data never do that; in fact, a lot of talk precedes the actual rendering of a recommendation. I had to ask myself the question: "What is all this talk accomplishing?"

At a superficial level, this question is partly answered by reference to the current movement in medicine to be "patient-centered" (Laine & Davidoff, 1996). This movement encompasses physician behaviors which favor fully informing patients about diagnosis, prognosis, and possible complications in treatment. Some of this informing behavior has been legally mandated, particularly in the area of informed consent to treatment (Laine & Davidoff, 1996). But from a social and linguistic point of view, there is clearly something else being accomplished by the talk, which relates to the overall sense that these visits are not just informative but are also persuasive.

Oncologists are trained in the art and science of treating cancer; they believe they know what is best for the patient from a medical point of view. Indeed, in contrast to a physician interviewed who believes he presents options evenly to patients, another highly respected oncologist discussed this aspect of his work with me. This second informant said his job is not just to present options, but to encourage his patients in a particular direction.

At the same time, the patient brings *her* understanding of her illness and her own concerns about possible further treatment. The discussions being studied here are aimed, theoretically, at informing patients about treatment options and finding out what the patient wants to do in light of that information. How does the doctor manage informing about the options while persuading the patient to take a particular course of action?

1.3 Expertise and Recommendations: Constructing Participant Roles

In cancer treatment, writing prescriptions for patients is not enough. Doctors must make relevant, believable, and persuasive the recommendations that they are giving, particularly in the face of potential patient resistance to those recommendations. To be both persuasive and to be persuaded involves, to some extent, the presentation and recognition of "expertise." In this volume I look at how expertise is constructed through talk; and how it is called on as a resource by both patients and doctors.

Some would argue that doctors are viewed, a priori, as experts in Western culture, and, most important, that we take their advice *because* they are doctors.[4] This stems from a traditional view of doctor-patient asymmetry, one which assumes doctors are powerful because they are knowledgeable while patients are not. But this static, simplistic view of power and expertise ignores the interactive work that goes on within a medical encounter to construct these relationships; they are not preordained role sets but are cooperatively achieved by the participants on a moment to moment basis. In this way, the current investigation is aligned with a trend in discourse studies away from a deterministic view of power and expertise and toward a more dynamic perception.

Other scholars working within a conversation analytic framework have taken a similar stance. Heath (1992), investigating the diagnostic phase of initial medical interviews in British general practice clinics, reveals how patients subordinate their knowledge to the doctor's by withholding replies to the announcement of a diagnosis or by designing their contributions so that they support the doctor's explanations. Thus, the asymmetry of the relationship is accomplished by both parties through their conversational practices in the moments of interaction.

In a similar clinical context in the Netherlands, ten Have (1991) demonstrates that patients can get their informational needs met by formulating their "ignorance" in medical matters. On occasions where they present concerns about their medical situation, patients may do so in a way that a response from the physician is not necessarily required (pp. 146-148). Thus patients are seen to present their questions as "ignorable." In a similar vein, in a U.S. general practice setting, Gill (1995) shows how patient causal explanations for their medical complaints can be reported as simple circumstances or events, not as explicitly linked to a health problem. Such reports can be attended to as news by the doctor and simply incorporated into the activity of information gathering. In this way, "doctors are provided with opportunities to avoid assessing what patients know about causation" (p. 196), without explicitly ignoring the patient altogether. In effect, patients present theories about the source of their illness in such a way that physicians can avoid those explanations as not medically relevant.

Finally, in a U.S. study of the ongoing medical relationships between physicians and parents of developmentally disabled children, Barton (1996) demonstrates how family members may structure the visit through their selection of topics and the development of those topics, presenting themselves and being treated as experts. Therefore, as Barton highlights "speakers actively negotiate desired roles and relationships within institutional discourse rather than passively act [them] out" (p. 303).

In sum, we are discovering the ways in which doctor-patient asymmetry is jointly accomplished and what the conversational mechanisms are that create and sustain that asymmetry. The current study examines this broader concern and in the process tries to understand the ways in which doctors persuade patients, by demonstrating how oncologist expertise is instantiated through talk-in-interaction. I work from the premise that doctors are not expert service providers simply because they carry specialized knowledge in their heads; rather, they are experts by virtue of the social practices which, in concert with patient actions, establish them as gatekeepers to knowledge and by the expertise/knowledge that they display or invoke in interaction. Expertise is not, therefore, simply a fact of professional preparation but is also a cooperatively constructed social phenomenon.

In addition to the joint accomplishment of physician expertise in medical settings, this study examines the interactive accomplishment of advice-giving. In institutional settings, it is clear that recommendations, advice, or their possible precursor the delivery of bad news are all interactionally achieved or failed. Research indicates that when doctors (or other health workers) provide information to their patients or clients, whether it is called "advice" or a "recommendation," acceptance of or resistance to the recommendations can be accounted for by the conversational actions of *both* participants.

In a study of recommendations in U.S. outpatient clinics, Costello (1990) shows that physicians first provide accounts for their recommendations and may subsequently modify them according to patient response. If the recommendation is met with silence, hesitation, or verbal displays of concern, the physician may move to modify and reformulate it (pp. 62-63).

Heritage and Sefi (1992) demonstrate that in British home health visits, failing to properly account for the advice given (i.e., giving advice "unilaterally" without justification), home health visitors risk meeting with advice resistance from their clients. In their data, unproblematic encounters are those in which the client/mother has in some way asked for advice, setting herself up, through the talk, as an advice recipient.

In support of Heritage and Sefi, Silverman, Bor, Miller, and Goldman (1991) conclude that advice that is "recipient designed" (Schegloff, 1972) renders the uptake of advice unproblematic. Based on both a conversation analysis and supplemental quantitative analyses, Silverman et al. find a correlation between the way that advice is set up or "given" by the counselor (in British AIDS counseling) and how it is received by the client.

Similarly, research by Maynard (1991b, 1992) demonstrates how, in a U.S. clinic for developmentally disabled children, clinicians use of a parent's perspective, elicited as an embedded feature in the course of news delivery, is instrumental in persuading that parent to align with the clinical position. Importantly, however, Maynard argues elsewhere (1991a) that researchers erroneously assume that "failure to communicate only means that a person has not exerted the effort to pack thoughts into words" (p. 160). His caution against assuming that "good" clinical interaction relies on "good message packaging" is clearly relevant. Research on the features of what constitutes smooth or problematic interaction is just beginning, and the insights gained will be extremely instructive.

Thus, the current study is intended as a contribution to this literature on recommendations, as well as to the previously mentioned literature on expertise—as I found them to be closely related concerns in the current data. Essentially, then, this book demonstrates how activities within the clinic visit create and maintain participant roles in the interaction as they move toward, and ultimately accomplish, the presentation, justification, and discussion of the recommendation for the patient's particular case.

The approach taken here is to import as little as possible into the data analysis and to notice what is made relevant by the participants through their verbal actions. In the remainder of this chapter, a review of the general literature on doctor-patient interaction distinguishes the major trends in the research and provides support for the conversation analytic framework used here. The review is intended both as a resource for those new to the field and as a backdrop for the methodological choices made in this study.

1.4 Review of Literature on Doctor-Patient Communication

All of the research reviewed here has taken verbal interaction as the starting point for understanding medical interaction. Roter and Hall (1992) discuss the centrality of talk in the practice of medicine, noting that it is "the main ingredient in medical care . . . the fundamental instrument by which the doctor-patient relationship is crafted and by which therapeutic goals are achieved" (p. 3). Though there is agreement that talk is at the center of the social, diagnostic, and therapeutic work of medicine, approaches for understanding that talk have varied substantially. Divergent theoretical and clinical concerns of many different fields have produced a wide range of important studies: Anthropologists, linguists, sociologists, public health professionals, and physicians themselves have all contributed to a better understanding of the patient-physician dynamic. So, at the risk of oversimplifying, but for ease of discussion, I divide the research that has not yet been touched on in this introduction into sociomedical research and discourse studies—two approaches that have relatively clear, though not impermeable methodological boundaries.

1.4.1 Sociomedical Studies of Medical Interaction

The earliest research approach to doctor-patient communication was based on the collection of interview or questionnaire data and, more recently, on methods that rely on the investigator to distill interactions into discrete codable behaviors. This type of research often presents findings in a quantitative, usually statistical, framework. Talk is the raw data for analysis, but the verbal interaction is usually not treated in its naturally occurring sequences. Rather, categories or types of interactional sequences (such as questions) or total amount of talk is quantified, usually in relation to demographic characteristics of interest.[5] I call this "sociomedical" research because the methodologies used are closest to traditional sociological approaches for understanding social phenomena.

Investigators in the sociomedical tradition were pioneers in the study of doctor-patient interaction. One of the first studies, conducted by a public health professional, was concerned with whether or not patients understood medical vocabulary regarding antepartum nutrition (Collins, 1955). That study, designed as a test of patient comprehension, was directed at improving patient care by better understanding whether or not physician talk was successfully transmitting information. This early concern, which remains with us today, revolves around medical outcomes: how to improve doctor-patient communication and thereby patient health behaviors. The most often studied areas in this line of research include patient satisfaction (Skipper, 1965; Smith, Polis, & Hadac, 1981; Buller & Buller, 1987; Hadlow & Pitts, 1991; Phillips, 1996) and patient compliance with treatment regimens (Davis, 1968; Svarstad, 1979; Steele, Jackson, & Guntmann, 1990[6]), the latter often related to patient understanding of medical information (Collins 1955; McKinlay, 1975; Bourhis, Roth, & MacQueen, 1989). This type of "quality of care" research has been concerned with information exchange in the medical setting, the premise being that aspects of communication, if improved, will lead to improved satisfaction for both physicians and patients (Korsch & Negrete, 1972; Roter & Hall, 1992).

In pursuit of improving communication and of better understanding what patients need in the medical setting, many points of entry to the problem have been tried, though with substantial methodological variability. The body of research is vast and at the same time rather disparate in terms of approaches and findings. Such a combination of ever- increasing output with ever-divergent methods has led to a challenging analytic situation. As Roter, Hall, and Katz (1988) observe in a review and meta-analysis of 61 of these quantitatively oriented investigations: "The field appears to be disorganized, with little sense of theoretical cohesiveness or rational progression" (p. 100).

Indeed, over the last 30 years, investigators have developed or applied an array of interaction analysis schemes which may or may not have been originally designed for observational study of medical interaction. Ong, DeHaes, Hoos, and Lammes (1995) identify 12 major interaction analysis schemes that have been used in the study of doctor-patient communication; in addition, researchers have developed their own unique systems, sometimes with little concern for matching coding category definitions or communication variables with prior studies (Roter et al., 1988). Thus, there has been a proliferation of terms with little attention to coherence among them, though some findings remain congruous across studies (e.g., female patients receive more total communication than do male patients; Hall, Roter, & Katz, 1988). For the reader who is interested in discerning the major findings of the quantitative studies of doctor-patient communication studies, two reviews and one meta-analysis help enormously in that regard (see Hall et al., 1988; Roter et al., 1988; Ong et al., 1995).

The advantage of the quantitative approaches to understanding medical interaction is that such approaches can quickly identify factors that may affect doctor-patient interaction (e.g., comprehensibility of medical terminology or aspects of patient satisfaction) and thus can alert clinicians to areas that require attention. However, from a communication point of view, they risk turning the talk into a "by-product" of the physician-patient relationship (West, 1984b, p. 34). When the verbal interactions are dissected and disembodied, yielding data which can then be broken down into codable, countable bits and pieces, talk is treated as an abstraction that supplants the participants' own orientations to their unfolding encounter. In the same way that laboratory and other "objective" data have come to supersede the patient's experience of their illness (Roter & Hall, 1992, pp. 3–5), until recently, the concomitant reduction of medical interaction into manageable chunks of data has come to supersede the realities of the talk itself. The process of coding talk may help characterize the actions of the participants in broad strokes, but the characterization is from the analyst's point of view, not the participant's. And though associations are generally found between sociodemographic factors and communication variables (as with the findings about females receiving more talk), determining causality remains an elusive goal (Hall et al., 1988). Because actual behaviors are lost in the system that is trying to render them comprehensible (see Frankel, 1984, esp. n. 1, for a compelling discussion of this issue), the question of causal relationship is difficult to approach.

Thus, the value of characterizing interaction from a quantitative perspective must be weighed against the necessary abstractness that such approaches introduce. Whether or not analytic categories are relevant to participant orientations to their own activities, as evidenced in the ongoing talk, must be continuously monitored. Schegloff (1993) convincingly presents possible constraints on quantitative research for understanding talk-in-interaction and persuasively argues for certain "conditions . . . under which it may be warrantably undertaken" (p. 100). This is not to say that quantitative and qualitative approaches cannot or should not complement one another. In fact, both social scientists and public health researchers have argued for the value of cross-methodological study of medical issues (Roter & Frankel, 1992; Verhoef & Casebeer, 1997). My point is simply that a principled approach to quantifying talk should take into account the participants' orientation to their activity, what they make relevant as members in the interaction. In that way, recurrent patterns of interactionally relevant items may present themselves as countable, and some kinds of comparative study may be possible.

1.4.2 Discourse Studies of Medical Interaction

In contrast to the proliferation of quantitative analyses of doctor-patient interactions, fewer studies have taken a qualitative approach to understanding the medical setting. In the late 1970s and early 1980s, several important studies appeared which took a discourse/linguistic/ethnographic approach to analyzing physician-patient interactions (e.g., Cicourel, 1981, 1983; Fisher, 1982, 1983, 1984; Mishler, 1984; Tannen & Wallat 1983; Todd, 1984). Though many of these investigators are doing "sociomedical" research, I refer to this second group as "discourse studies" of medical interaction because the analysis stays closer to examining stretches of conversation.[7] However, in contrast to studies in a CA framework of that same period (e.g., Frankel, 1983, 1984; West, 1983, 1984a, 1984b) the discourse studies begin with an assumption that interaction is shaped by sociopolitical forces, belief, or knowledge systems.

Many of the discourse studies of medical interaction have focused on understanding the asymmetrical relationship between doctor and patient (though one of the early studies, Tannen and Wallet [1983], is concerned with how a pediatrician manages the competing tasks of addressing multiple audiences). The early research is concerned not only with understanding and improving doctor-patient communication but also with demonstrating that language practices in the medical setting embody larger sociopolitical relations, most notably power and gender. The analytic stance of many of these investigations is often one in which interaction is viewed as being directed by actors outside the talk; social constructs are given a central, taken-for-granted role in the discourse.

Among those taking a discourse/ethnographic approach to understanding medical communication, Cicourel was one of the first, building on a broader interest in the intersection of language, meaning, and social interaction (Cicourel, 1974). In medical interactions, Cicourel's concern has been with asymmetry of communicative power in the physician-patient relationship and the problem of miscommunication (Cicourel, 1981, 1983). He has focused attention on physician "recoding" of patient talk as formulated in doctors' medical reports of ambulatory care visits.

Investigating the difference between doctor-patient communication (what is said) and the information that is distilled from those verbal encounters and written up as texts destined for colleagues, Cicourel concludes that competing belief systems and different forms of literacy contribute to miscommunication in the medical setting. He further argues that physician-patient interaction is a "microcosm" of the communicative complexities of society at large in which members possess different symbolic systems for interacting with each other, especially in professional-layperson situations (Cicourel, 1983, p. 238). In a sense, the competing symbolic systems are seen as leading to miscommunication, not the participants themselves, who simply embody those systems.

Similarly, Mishler's concern with humane medical care leads to an analysis in which there is a struggle between the voice of the patient's "lifeworld" and the "voice of medicine." As such, patient explanations for their ill health become disrupted and fragmented, with the more powerful voice of medicine imposing order (Mishler, 1984, p. 190). Studies by Fisher (1983,

1984) and Todd (1984) also argue that the doctor's authority within the medical institution structures the discourse. They maintain that because patient and doctor share a common social order, their view of the medical relationship is also shared and influences the exchange of information and the process of decision making.

In these studies, asymmetry of the physician-patient relationship is seen either as shaping their discourse practices or as reflected in them. By isolating a particular discourse structure or speech act, these investigators conclude that its distribution or use is explained by social forces at work in the setting. For example, Todd (1984) maintains that physician power is reflected in the skewed distribution of questions and directives and by topic control. Mishler (1984) examined and also highlighted the different questioning practices and topic control as indicators of physician dominance in medical encounters; more recently, Ainsworth-Vaughn (1992) expanded the notion of topic control by studying topic transitions. She finds a statistically significant interaction among physician gender and the type of topic transition activity (with female physicians utilizing a higher ratio of "reciprocal" to "unilateral" topic transitions).

Though talk is at the center of the analysis in these discourse studies, and analyses are supported with transcriptions of audiorecorded visits, the "endogenous orientations" of the interactants (Schegloff, 1997) is less a focus of study than broader conceptual concerns. Discourse, in this view, is seen as an effect of institutional rules and socially predetermined roles. The participants' agency is obscured in the shadow of contextual features that the analyst brings to the investigation. By presupposing that belief systems, power, and gender are relevant to an interaction, investigators find interesting associations between types of linguistic behavior and social roles, but they risk missing *how* the participants are accomplishing their roles through *coordinated* social activity and how they invoke roles to accomplish activities in particular moments of interaction (see Halkowski, 1990, for an excellent example of the latter approach in the context of U.S. congressional hearings).

Rather than presupposing what the roles and beliefs of the participants might be, one of the aims of the current study, along with other CA studies, is to look at medical discourse for what the participants are accomplishing with their talk, and how they are doing so.

Ainsworth-Vaughn (1994) exemplifies a similar direction in discourse studies. She examines rhetorical questions and how they are used by both patients and doctors as a resource for creating ambiguity in medical interactions. In her analysis of ongoing doctor-patient relationships, ambiguity functions for both patients and physicians to temper otherwise threatening acts. Physicians use it to mitigate "their necessary violations of patients' personal and discourse rights" (p. 210) during, for example, the physical exam. Patients also use ambiguity (as embodied in rhetorical questions) to mitigate face-threatening acts (defined, for example, as questions directly posed to doctors or criticism of the doctor). This more complex view of "power" is one that allows for the agency of both participants in the interaction and examines how each interactant both exercises control and defers to the other. It is not so much that there is reciprocity or equal distribution of control over the event (Ainsworth-Vaughn, 1994, p. 195) but that both doctor and patient deploy resources of everyday talk for asserting different forms of control in medical relationships that have developed over time.

In conclusion, along with the conversation analytic research reviewed in the introduction to this chapter, it is clear that new attention is being brought to the study of the interactional dynamics of medical settings, particularly to the concerns of power and expertise and the associated activity of advice-giving. Quantitative studies of medical interaction have provided important insights, which continue to be fleshed out through detailed analyses of actual talk. By remaining alert to the observable orientations of the participants themselves, and by constraining the analysis so that those actions and orientations are at the center of the investigation, researchers will contribute greatly to understanding how a patient and a doctor interact in moments that are enormously consequential for both of them.

1.5 Outline of the Book

In chapter 2, I examine the theoretical background supporting the CA approach and describe my method for working with the data in this study. Details about data collection are included, as well as an overview of the study population.

In chapter 3, the overall structure of the recommendation visit is analyzed from a CA perspective, and I demonstrate how the component activities make these interactions identifiable not only as medical encounters but also as different from medical visits in general medicine clinics. I also show how the details of the talk maintain these visits as "service encounters" or as legitimate forums for the giving and receiving of advice.

After looking at the overall organization of the visit, chapter 4 examines the ways in which the roles of "expert" and "novice" are instantiated and deployed in these medical encounters. Here I explore how doing persuasion is related to establishing relative expertise. This chapter helps answer the question, "What is all this talk doing?"

Finally, after establishing how the interactional format is achieved and how identities are displayed, chapter 5 turns to the recommendation itself. All the talk that has preceded has been contributing to the participants' ability to arrive at this point. At the moment of the recommendation, they are engaged in the central purpose of the visit, and we will look at the particularities of that event in terms of the "patient's work" and the "doctor's work." The dilemma to be managed by the participants revolves around the patient's job of staying focused on her personal view of the risks and benefits of treatment and the doctor's job of promoting treatment based on statistical notions of risk for the general population. The doctor maintains a balance between not making any guarantees while still promoting his or her view of what is best for the patient.

By no means is the analysis presented here to be considered "the last word" on this data; the process of unpacking and understanding any stretch of naturally occurring talk is a nearly never-ending adventure. However, this study is intended to encourage further qualitative study of cancer treatment recommendations, since it is in the moments of talk that the oncologist and patient establish who they are and come to an understanding of what their visit is about. If we are to better comprehend the dynamics of talk and medicine in interaction, then we must begin by looking at how doctors and patients work through, on a moment to moment basis, the concerns that each brings to the encounter.

2

Analytic Approach

2.1 Conversation Analysis: A Justification

The methodology adopted for this study is conversation analysis. Evolving out of ethnomethodology, conversation analysis (CA) accounts for the verbal and coordinated nonverbal behaviors that participants use moment to moment to create, maintain, and re-create the social world. The advantage of using a CA methodology is that it privileges naturally occurring spoken interaction in a way that constrains the analyst from introducing "unsubstantiated intuitions" into an analysis (Levinson, 1983, p. 295). To fully understand this claim, a brief discussion of the theoretical foundations of conversation analysis in order.

Ethnomethodology developed within sociology as a reaction against prevailing deterministic views of social behavior. The conceptual framework was first elaborated by Garfinkel (1967) and later by Garfinkel and Sacks (1970). Garfinkel incorporated a phenomenological point of view into his approach to understanding social behavior. He asserted that we interpret our world based on patterns whose validity we assume until compelled to question them (Heritage, 1984, p. 77). From this, Garfinkel developed a key insight about the importance of observable patterns as enacted and enactable, as "do-able" elements of social interaction. One could pass as a particular gender or pass as a member of some ethnic group simply by "doing" what that category of person does (Garfinkel, 1967). In other words, commonsense categorical labels do not precede people but are constituted of observable behaviors, both verbal and otherwise.

Garfinkel proposed his theory in light of a series of real-world "breaching experiments." Beginning first with the game of tick-tack-toe, Garfinkel had his students engage friends and strangers in the game but had the student break a particular rule (by, for example, erasing the opponent's moves). Students then noted the responses. Behaviors fell into two basic categories: those that tried to normalize the event as part of a joke or as the experimenter's introduction of new rules for tick-tack-toe and those that demanded some kind of explanation. The former abandoned the interpretive framework of tick-tack-toe, treating it as some other "legal" activity—like playing a practical joke; the latter group, which tried to make sense of the breach in terms of the normal tick-tack-toe framework, showed they were disturbed by the breach and required an account or explanation to make sense of the experience.

Later, more difficult real-life experiments were devised in which student experimenters ask subjects (who were friends) to clarify commonplace remarks (e.g., "flat tire") in the course of some ordinary conversation. Again the reactions were carefully noted by the student experimenters. In doing this experiment, they uncovered a requirement or "rule" of conversation: that interlocutors supply background knowledge to make sense of the ongoing talk. When this rule was broken by the students asking for explanations of mundane objects, the sanctioning of the behavior was rapid and powerful (Heritage, 1984, p. 81). This was evident through the explanations or accounts sought by the subjects.

With these and other experiments, Garfinkel was able to show that stable patterns of social activity were the product of choices made by social actors who orient to "rules" of conduct which they attribute to one another, and in terms of which they hold one another accountable. The sense of "rule" for Garfinkel is not "an internalized norm of what is proper or desirable, but rather as constitutive of what perceivable events are, of 'what is going on here'" (Heritage, 1984, p. 83). In other words, it is not that a moral or sacred trust is being broken when activities are breached in this way but, rather, that social organization disintegrates because the sense of *what kind of event* is unfolding starts to break down. These "rules" allow us to recognize activities in terms of discernible patterns—though patterns of social activity are usually not consciously perceived by participants until there is some breach. In phone conversations, for example, we do not notice that our interlocutor is continually providing continuers (or "back channels") unless he or she stops doing so, and then we suddenly find ourselves asking, "Are you there?"

Because the fabric of social interaction is so finely woven, and so automatic, to get an understanding of it requires very close attention to the details. For this reason, the ethnomethodological (and related CA) approach "is characterized by strict and parsimonious structuralism . . . emphasis is on the data and the patterns recurrently displayed therein" (Levinson, 1983, p. 295). From this point of view of perceived patterning, the "context" of any bit of talk is not a free-standing or preexisting phenomenon which somehow "shapes" an interaction. Rather, participants work to create and maintain a context of shared understandings during the course of their encounters by orienting to (or not) the displayed orientations of their interlocutor: "It is not satisfactory to describe or interpret a setting by reference to rules or standards which are external to, or independent of, the ways in which the characteristics of the setting are recognized, used, produced, and talked about by the settings members" (Heritage, 1984, p. 133).

In this way, the analyst working in a CA framework is constrained from intuiting intentions on the part of participants; the theory is that participants themselves will demonstrate, or display through their responses and actions, anything that is relevant to their interaction.

Building on Garfinkel's ethnomethodological foundation, Sacks initiated conversation analysis as a form of ethnomethodological work, designed to "keep a grip" on the primary data of the social world (Heritage, 1984, p. 235). Whatever resources participants have at their disposal for making sense of their world should theoretically also be available to us as analysts of their interaction.

Conversation analysis is, then, a methodology grounded in the data of naturally occurring talk, and pays attention to the observable actions and orientations of the participants themselves. Sacks et al. (1974) originally proposed that talk is orderly, its shape in any instance reflecting particularized application of general, context-free interactional mechanisms or rules. This has been clearly demonstrated using CA methodology across a wide variety of settings and cultures (e.g., Atkinson & Drew, 1979, courtrooms; Moerman, 1988, legal proceedings in Thailand; Schegloff, 1992, news interviews; Zimmerman, 1992, emergency calls). Turn types and turn allocation can be deployed to instantiate many different conversational activities and speaker roles: It is not necessary to presuppose conversational identities to make sense of some stretch of talk.

By looking closely at the details of talk, such as turn types, hesitations, overlaps, laughter, and prosody, in addition to the more traditional objects of analysis such as lexicon and sentence structure, the current study takes account of as much of the verbal data as was available to the participants in the interaction. Though the transcription process is "motivated" (Ochs, 1979) by the perspective that as much of the detail as possible should be incorporated, the analysis itself is not hypothesis driven. That is, I do not begin with the assumption that doctors talk more or that patients interrupt less or that doctors are powerful and patients are not. Rather, by carefully transcribing the interaction, I am attempting to get at the orderliness of their talk which itself instantiates their displayed orientation to the activity under way. I will show, for example, that what makes one speaker a "doctor" and another a "patient" is not inherent to their persons or simply a matter of the education they may have had access to; expertise and training must be displayed and deployed and sought after. Further, the delivery of the recommendation is not an isolated unidirectional event but is formulated as part of the ongoing, sequential organization of speaker contributions.

2.2 Data Collection

The data for this study consisted of 22 audiotaped conversations ranging from 9 to 58 minutes. Though audiotaped data preclude the analysis of nonverbal interaction, some very recent and important insights about advice-giving have come from settings in which only audiotaping was allowed. Heritage and Sefi (1992) rely on audio-recorded visits by home health visitors, as do Silverman et al. (1991) for their analysis of safe sex advice in AIDS clinics. So, although video data are certainly preferable, they are not always obtainable. Nonetheless, the findings of the current study could be augmented and enriched should visual records of oncology clinic visits become available.

Each of the encounters in this data set is between a woman who has undergone surgery for breast cancer, the friends and family who may have accompanied her to the office visit, and an oncologist. The conversations were collected at two prestigious oncology centers which are incorporated into large teaching hospitals. Twenty-one of the audiotapes were loaned to me by Laura Siminoff. As described in Siminoff (1987), she relied on a sequential sample of patients for her study. This means that each woman entering the clinic over a 16-month period ($n = 107$) was asked if she would participate in the research. Ninety-three percent ($n = 100$) of those patients approached for her study consented to have their visit with the oncologist audiotaped while Siminoff or her assistant was in the room. The data for the current study, then, are drawn primarily from Siminoff's sequential, nonrandom sample of those 100 visits. The subsample of Siminoff's data used here was chosen neither randomly nor sequentially. I listened to all of Siminoff's original tapes and chose 21 of them for my study. The selection was motivated by the clarity of the audiotape and the age and race of the subject. I tried to get a cross-section of ages and races within the confines of audiotape quality. The additional audiotape in the sample was recorded by me during informal observations at an oncology center at a large teaching hospital.

Prior to discovering the existence of Siminoff's data set, I had begun ethnographic observations at the oncology center. These observations lasted for 6 weeks, usually 3 hours for one or two afternoons per week. The clinic specializes in treating breast problems using a team approach, so I was able to observe the medical oncologists, radiation oncologists, and surgeons who meet with patients at various stages in their breast cancer treatment. During this time I was able to participate in all aspects of the doctors' visits with the patients. My observation day began by standing with the doctors as they reviewed and discussed the charts of the patients they would be seeing that afternoon, accompanying doctors to the examination rooms, and sitting in the room during the consultation (following patient verbal consent). I generally did not follow up with patients afterward as my presence was considered a student observation and not a research study approved by the Institutional Review Board. I did, however, follow up the visit with the doctors to ask any questions that may have arisen for me during the medical encounter.

2.3 Analytic Procedures

I began this study by conducting observations and interviews at a clinic specializing in "breast problems" housed in a large teaching hospital. As will become apparent, however, I do not draw directly on that information for my analysis. The observations were primarily to establish a rapport with the oncologists at the clinic so that I could eventually propose a more formalized study and begin collecting audiotape data. I was also able to observe the setting in which Siminoff's tapes were made and to interview one of the oncologists with whom she worked. These observations helped me to have a visual sense of where the recommendation visits took place, usual proximity of the doctor and patient, any visual aids (e.g., blackboards and notepads) that were available, how they tended to be used, and so on.

Although this visual picture was helpful for me and may have influenced me in my listening, it does not play a central role in this work.

There is a lively debate among discourse and conversation analysts as to the role of ethnographic observations in analyzing talk-in-interaction (see Duranti & Goodwin, 1992, for an excellent volume devoted to exploring this topic.) Cicourel (1992) argues that ethnographic detail is essential for situating talk within an institutional context. And although I agree that such detail provides a certain texture and richness that is satisfying for readers, I do not believe that such detail is truly essential for understanding a stretch of talk. In the current study, I was faced with understanding 21 audio-recorded visits (from Siminoff's data) for which I had virtually no ethnographic background, never having met the patients or the doctors. I did have some medical information for the patients, including their age, stage of disease, and the treatment option they eventually chose. (This information is also provided for the reader in appendix A.)

Having very little information on the participants was quite freeing. The situation forced me to hear only what the participants heard, to evoke only the information that was made available by the participants themselves. For the tape that I collected, I was familiar with the oncologist and knew his standing in the hospital and community, but I knew nothing of the patient. I was confronted with a kind of exercise in "audiotape archaeology" and never felt the need to know "more" than what the participants were offering to each other. My concern was not to situate these encounters within a larger social or institutional context; my concern was to identify how the participants in these visits created a local context through their talk and actions, how they created and maintained ongoing social and medical activities within the fleeting moments of their interaction.

Most of the work for the current study involved the transcription and analysis of the 22 audiotapes. Transcription conventions were based on Jefferson (1974) and appear in appendix B. The central analytic work began with listening to the audiotapes several times and keeping a log of the activities and talk that I noticed in a very general way. After listening to the tapes and noting some general areas of interest (overall organization, display of expertise, patient resistance to recommendations), I began to transcribe each tape in detail. The transcriptions were accomplished one tape at a time, so that I followed each interaction in detail from beginning to end. After doing half the audiotapes in this way, I felt confident about leaving certain portions of the tapes only roughly transcribed and focused my efforts on those portions of the interactions that concerned me most. Specifically, I stopped transcribing the medical-history-taking portion of the tapes and worked only on the openings (elicitation of patient concerns) and the portion in which the recommendation was delivered. It seemed to me that these were the two most consequential areas in the interactions and the least well described elsewhere. The standard medical interview (the medical history taking) is most often focused on and has been carefully described elsewhere (Byrne & Long, 1976; Mishler, 1984). Nonetheless, I will cover medical history taking in my analysis in as much as participant orientations to it are important for understanding how roles are constituted within the interaction.

Once the tapes were transcribed, I began the work of doing line-by-line analysis of a single consultation (Patient 2 and Doctor 2). I worked through that interaction in an "unmotivated" way (Sacks, 1984), assuming as little as possible about the participants and what they were doing. For example, I did not even assume the sex of the participants; voice quality (pitch) was the first indication of the speaker's sex, and as information was revealed about medical history (e.g., undergoing hysterectomy or giving birth to children), I was able to categorize one speaker as female. I relied only on voice quality to assign a sex to each doctor but recognized them as doctors (or near counterparts) because they had special rights to perform a physical examination on the woman, and she showed no objection.

The purpose of this exercise in audiotape archaeology was just to hear the talk for what it was, to notice how the participants responded to what was said and done, not how I, as the analyst, was responding. Approaching the data in this way led to insights which I then carried to other audiotapes in the data set. I began to look for recurrent patterns and also took note of problematic or disrupted patterns. In this way, the analysis took shape "on the back of the single case" (Schegloff, 1993).

2.4 Subjects

Siminoff's female subjects are distributed in age ranges similar to the national distribution of women with breast cancer at the time of data collection (Siminoff, 1987). Combining the sample of data she loaned to me and my own audio-recording, nine different physicians (one female, Doctor 6) are included in the data set. The patients range in age from 22 to 73. White and African American women are represented, in both older and younger age brackets. Readers interested in further detail should refer to appendix A where demographic and medical characteristics of each patient are provided.

3

Phased Organization of the Adjuvant Therapy Visit

Medical visits are characteristically organized into a series of activity phases corresponding to specific medical and social tasks to be accomplished. In an analysis of more than 1,800 general medical practice encounters, Byrne and Long (1976) distinguish the following six phases: *relating to the patient* (conversational openings), *discovering the reason for the visit, conducting verbal and/or physical exams, considering the patient's condition* (presenting diagnostic information to the patient), *advising treatment or further testing,* and *termination* (conversational closings). These findings, based on an analysis of physician verbal behavior, have not been substantially revised since that pioneering analysis (Heath, 1992; Mishler, 1984). Heath (1992) does refine our understanding of the diagnostic phase, but the essential format originally outlined by Byrne and Long (1976) remains intact.

The medical visits analyzed for the current study adhere to the general six-phase framework, though when examined in detail, the workings within some of the phases are rather different from general medical visits. From the outset, for example, *discovering the reason for the visit* is a seemingly redundant exercise in these encounters. As is discussed, oncologists are quite aware ahead of time of the patient's reason for the visit, and the patient is fully aware of the nature and seriousness of her condition. The question for the analyst then becomes: "What is this talk doing here?" Further, patients are afforded extended turns in this initial phase, setting this particular type of medical visit distinctly apart from general medical encounters in which patient contributions are often cut short within, on average, the first 18 seconds of the visit (Beckman & Frankel, 1984).

As discussions of adjuvant therapy for breast cancer have not been fully described elsewhere in terms of component activities or turn organization, this chapter examines those phenomena. The analysis reveals the overall structure of these oncology clinic interactions and shows specifically how the shape of the turns (who speaks and when) and the content (what is attended to as an appropriate contribution) construct these interactions as institutional service encounters which are legitimate occasions for giving and receiving recommendations.

We begin with an overview of the activity phases of the clinic visit as evidenced by the participants' orientation to that organization and then discuss the relevance of particular activities: the elicitation of disease status, which provides a point of departure for the recommendation; the transition into, and a brief look at, the collection of medical history; then finally oncologists' resistance to "troubles-telling," which maintains the service orientation of these encounters. The recommendation itself, and patient response to the recommendation, is discussed in chapter 5.

3.1 The Main Activity Phases Preceding the Recommendation

Each consultation in the current data contains four major topic areas, each representing a set of tasks to be accomplished. These topic areas roughly match the central phases of the general medicine clinic visit as described by Byrne and Long (1976), though each is elaborated in some unique ways. The described phases are not simply analytic entities to help outsiders make sense of the data; they are oriented to by the participants themselves, which is what makes the phases our concern. Following is a synopsis of the main activity phases in terms of topical content and turn types and turn allocation mechanisms that are prevalent. Phase numbering corresponds to that of prior research, so, leaving aside for the moment conversational openings and closings (Phases 1 and 6) we begin with Phase 2.

Phase 2. Elicitation of Concerns

The doctor elicits the patient's orientation to the office visit; the patient tells her story and frames her concerns/asks questions. Subtopics/tasks within this phase can include retrospection (events leading up to the discovery of the tumor), establishing current state of emotional and physical health, and establishing patient's understanding of her condition.

Turn description: The doctor asks brief open-ended questions of the patient and then cooperates as a recipient in the patient's extended turns. This is in contrast to general medicine clinic visits, where it has been shown that 69% of patients are interrupted during their description of the reason for their visit and the talk immediately gets focused by the doctor onto a particular problem, often the first mentioned (Beckman & Frankel, 1984).

Phase 3. Collection of Medical History
The doctor collects standard medical and demographic information by questioning the patient, during which time there is an elaboration of any health concerns that may be relevant to cancer treatment. Subtopics/tasks include enumerating any noncancer medications, chronic illnesses or complaints, surgical history relative to reproductive health, family history of cancer, current family support system and occupational status.

Turn description: Questions which elicit factual information or yes/no answers are posed by the doctor and met with short answers from the patient. Patient questions tend to be dispreferred during this phase.

Phase 4. Physical Examination
The patient undergoes a brief physical exam, focusing primarily on the surgical site. This phase was not audio-recorded.

Phase 5. The Recommendation
The doctor provides information relevant to prognosis and treatment options; the patient asks questions. Subtopics/tasks include establishing the relevance of diagnostic information (lymph node involvement, tumor size), clarifying the mechanisms of metastasis, enumerating the side effects of adjuvant therapies, explaining experimental protocols, and making a treatment recommendation.

Turn description: The doctor has extended turns in which the patient cooperates as a recipient. Both doctors and patients pose questions during this phase.

These phases most often appear in the order presented. If there is any variation in the order it is that information usually appearing in phase 5 may be introduced early in the encounter by the oncologist and then returned to after the physical examination. The doctors display an orientation to the order as outlined here by announcing upcoming topics/activities and by occasionally resisting patient attempts to move outside or ahead of the current activity. It is this oriented-to aspect of the oncologist's actions, discussed further in section 3.2, that reveals these phases and subtopics as tasks to be accomplished within the time span of the adjuvant therapy visit.

3.2 Physician Orientation to the Phases

In this section we see how the oncologist has a set of tasks to accomplish, and how he or she mentions the activities, pursues them, and at times resists the patient's attempts to move off of the task/topic under way. This is evidence not only of orientation to an agenda but perhaps more important, the deployment of the agenda as a resource for managing the conversation such that certain issues or topics are delayed. For the current study, this aspect of physician behavior is critical for understanding how oncologists manage and display their institutional roles as experts and gatekeepers to information.

The oncologists in these data, not the patients, characteristically mention specific activities to be accomplished, or "agenda" items. These correspond generally to the descriptors I have given to the individual phases: elicitation of concerns, taking medical history, physical examination, treatment recommendation. When the agenda unfolds unproblematically, it is treated as a simple projection of future activity without resistance from the patient. Thus, though the patient shows no orientation to an agenda, she can be seen to cooperate in the doctor's control of the visit. The following two excerpts (see appendix B for transcription conventions) are examples of unproblematic movement through the oncologists's agenda:

Excerpt 1

102	PT 27		. . . I but I just wanted someone else's
103			opinion.
104	DR 4		Okay. Let's do this then, um let me just catch up
105		A→	quickly with ya about how ya been feelin. I'd
106		B→	like to examine ya briefly. and then we'll
107		C→	leave plenty a time to talk about these (.)
108			*things*. I can give ya straightforward answers
109			*today for these questions.*
110	PT 27		Well that's what I want.

Excerpt 2

119	DR 2		Well what I thought we'd do is uh
120	PT 2		((sniff))
121	DR 2	B→	I'd examine you and the::n we'd talk a bit
122		C→	about (.) what it means to have a couple of
123			lymph nodes positive. in breast cancer.
124			What we know about that. (.) And what it
125			means (.) in t- in terms of lo::ng term
126			outlook, (.) an::d what kind of treatments (.)
127			are given in order to try to improve (the)
128			outlook. *Keh?* (.) I'd like to do that after I
129			take a look at you *n examine ya*.
130	PT 2		mm
131	DR 2		Kay? so why don't I have you step in there
132			put a gown on . . .

The doctor's orientation to a preferred order of events is clear in the preceding examples. In excerpt 1, the doctor goes on record (arrow A) as having a preference for hearing the patient's concerns. Then, in both excerpts, the doctor mentions a preference for first doing a physical exam (arrows B) and then speaking to the concerns raised by the patient (arrows C). These examples are typical of 66% ($n = 14$) of the cases in these data in which the physical examination is invoked as part of the work to be accomplished during the visit. (Cases in which no physical examination takes place include one particularly distressed patient and two patients of the eight patients who were referred for second opinions.) These early and explicit statements of the doctor's plans, as exemplified in excerpts 1 and 2, are quite frequent and serve as evidence that the oncologist has certain tasks to perform in the context of the visit and that the patient is invited to cooperate in that order of events.

Further evidence for a preference for a particular order of topics or activities is apparent in the next two excerpts. In what follows we see that the doctor treats the patient's contributions or questions as not relevant to the current activity. In this way, the doctor invokes the potentiality of the agenda to serve as a postponement from, at the moment, an unanswerable or dispreferred question. Marking the patient's question as in some way "out of order" can be used as a resource for managing the direction of the talk. Though the medical agenda being adhered to by the oncologists is not particularly unusual, what is noticeable is how it is used as a resource, being invoked to delay or manage the sequence of activities and information as we see in excerpts 3 and 4.

In excerpt 3, the oncologist attempts to redirect the talk as the patient attempts to move outside the confines of the activity at hand. The doctor has been covering general medical history and demographics (phase 3 topics) and has just asked the patient if she works outside the home. She says that she has worked as a consultant. At line 165 the patient then says:

Excerpt 3

165	PT 59	/That's/ another question when I go through
166		treatment am I going to be able to work.
167	DR 7	Well lemme- what I plan on doing (.) i:s I
168		wanna (.) get this information from you, I do
169		want to examine you briefly just to (.) check
170		things over, and then we'll go through the uh.
171		The answer to that would be: yes uh:::: . . .

Here, at line 165, the patient refers back (with the word "another") to the doctor's initial invitation that she tell him about her concerns; that is, the reason for visit (covered in phase 2). In terms of the proposed outline of phases 2–5, the patient's question, "Will I be able to work?" is out of order here. If there is a canonical format being oriented to, the phase of the encounter in which the patient's concerns were elicited (phase 2) has since passed; further, the participants are currently engaged in the collection of medical and demographic information (phase 3). Apparently, the patient is not orienting to the component phases in the same way that the doctor is. The "out of orderness" of the patient's question is revealed as such by the doctor's response (lines 167–170) in which he displays a dispreferred stance toward the patient's question. The "well" which launches his utterance is a token often associated with nonaffiliative or dispreferred responses; that is, it introduces some form of disagreement to come (Pomerantz, 1984). And the doctor's emphasis on the first-person pronoun in that first utterance is implicitly in contrast with some other person's plan (Maynard, 1992, p. 356, note 3). He is apparently contrasting what *he* the doctor wants to do with what the patient might want to do. He significantly delays his response to the question until line 171.

In essence, by overtly stating his plan of action for the next few moments and by delaying his response to the patient's question, the doctor is moving to disallow the question at this moment. In fact, after providing a brief comment on whether or not the patient can return to work, the doctor proceeds to ask the husband what kind of work he does. The agenda is reset to the point where it was broken off in-as-much as demographic information is being collected, albeit from the patient's husband. Clearly, the doctor is determining what is a locally relevant contribution; these sorts of delaying and side-stepping actions are never initiated by patients in this data. Asymmetrical control of the agenda achieved in this way is thus an observable feature of these interactions.

In the next excerpt, we see how the oncologist quickly moves to shift out of the topic that he himself has initiated once the patient raises a concern within that topic. Again, it is clear that the doctor's control of the agenda goes relatively unchallenged. This visit began with eliciting some medical information (phase 3 topics) and then moved to a general discussion about chemotherapy (phase 5 topic). So in this case the doctor himself has initiated the phase 5 discussion earlier than normal. When the patient makes a topically coherent contribution, framed as a question about alternatives to chemotherapy, the oncologist moves to stem the discussion.

Excerpt 4

DR 10		. . . ih it's kind of (.) therapy to prevent the
		problem instead of treating the problem after it
		comes up.
		(1.5)
PT 96		Well (is there) other treatment besides this type
		though? Or doctor [Mc] he explained to me- he told
		me, (1.0) that (.) he- if I needed it, he wouldn't give
		me chemotherapy or, /I could take a pill./
		(2.0)
DR 10		There- right there are other, uh, not all of
		adjuvant therapy is chemotherapy. Some of it is is
		hormonal therapy [(fortunately).
PT 96		[Right.
		(2.0)
DR 10	→	Why don't I examine you though and then we can
		talk more about
PT 96		Okay.
DR 10		about what we definitely would recommend in in
		your case.
PT 96		Okay.
DR 10		Okay?
PT 96		mm?

234	DR 10	There should be a gown for you in the back room
235		there.
236	PT 96	All right.

The patient's question is answered in lines 221–223. Her uptake of that answer ("right") in line 224 followed by a 2-second pause indicates the floor is open for either speaker to self-select (Sacks et al., 1974). The doctor takes a turn to introduce the activity of the physical exam but projects that there will be more talk about the patient's specific case after that. His use of the word "though" (line 226) indicates a contrast: Rather than further their discussion of types of therapies at this point, he would like to establish a different order, that is, proceed to the physical examination and take up specific concerns later on. The patient displays no resistance to that plan (lines 228, 231, 233, 236).

In this excerpt, the patient raises an implicit resistance to chemotherapy by asking a question about alternative treatments she claims to have heard about from another doctor. Though this is a relevant contribution at this sequential point in terms of the *content* of their current discussion, and the doctor answers the query, he clearly moves to delay this seemingly relevant topic. Even though the patient does not pursue the matter further, the doctor explicitly asks to put it off until after the exam. In this way, he displays not only that he is managing the agenda for the visit but also that this was not his final word on the subject. He thereby instantiates his role as gatekeeper to information that the patient has come in search of.

What excerpts 1 through 4 indicate is that the oncologists in these interactions invoke an agenda of activities and topics which they want to get through in a particular order, an order made explicit as exemplified in excerpts 1 and 2. Invoking the agenda (as we see in excerpts 3 and 4) works to postpone patient initiated topics. Indeed, the doctor's contributions in excerpts 3 and 4 retroactively mark the patient's questions as in some way "out of order." In this way the agenda can be used as a resource for managing the direction of the talk. Unresisted by the patient, these moments ratify the doctor as the gatekeeper of information.

3.3 Establishing a "Ticket of Entry" in Phase 2

Roughly 75% ($n = 16$) of the consultations begin with the oncologist asking the patient to describe her reason for coming to the clinic that day and asking what questions, if any, the patient has. The four remaining cases, in which there is no elicitation of the patient's reason for the visit, are discussed in the notes to this chapter. These few cases differ in specific ways that are related to the larger context of the patient's contact with the doctor thus far, technical failure of the tape recorder, or just a slight variation in the opening sequence.[1]

Eliciting the patient's reason for visit is a standard opening for general medical interviews. As Beckman and Frankel (1984) point out, this is prescribed as proper procedure by medical textbooks, and general practitioners are trained to do this. Unless the patient has come for a follow-up visit, the general practice physician needs the patient to describe the impetus for the visit. Patient-provided information allows the doctor to form a hypothesis regarding diagnosis; he or she then proceeds to test the hypothesis through further questioning, physical examination, and lab tests (Beckman & Frankel, 1984).

In the current data, however, the invitation to disclose a reason for the visit has special significance. The physician essentially knows why the patient has been referred, and the patient is aware that she has a life-threatening illness; there is no need for diagnosis. These physicians are medical oncologists, a specialty that entails prescription and management of chemical agents for cancer treatment following surgery. Thus almost any person having a clinic appointment with a medical oncologist is involved in a component activity of someone in or near the category of "cancer patient." More important, the doctor usually has the patient's full medical record and has read it, or at least skimmed it, by the time the consultation begins. This is evident in the talk itself as well as from the observations I made. And doctors often mention to the patient that they have read the medical record prior to their meeting. I propose, then, that establishing the patient's reason for the visit is, on the face of it, an apparently superfluous activity. Yet it occurs in nearly all the visits and therefore requires careful attention because it is being treated by the participants as one aspect of the work to be done.

By asking the patient's perspective on her condition, one might claim that the doctor is simply following a usual habit established during medical training. But it will become apparent that there is a specific function associated with the invitation to disclose a reason for the clinic visit. I propose that the activity of soliciting the patient's assessment of her state of health provides a "ticket of entry" (Heritage & Sefi, 1992, p. 412; Sacks, 1972) into the job at hand—namely describing treatment options and making a recommendation for further treatment. The original conception of a ticket of entry as described by Sacks (1972) was to account for the use of certain devices by children to ensure entry into conversations with adults.

Essentially, the argument ran that children have "limited rights" to speak. Children use forms such as "guess what?"—a recipient-designed query which elicits a "what?" response from the adult—to gain entry into a topic with an adult speaker.

Heritage and Sefi (1992) refer to the "ticket-of-entry problem" in their work about home health visitors in Britain who conduct obligatory visits to new mothers within the first weeks *post partum*. Because in this context the HVs have "no practical nursing responsibilities" the ticket-of-entry problem is raised: "the issue of what the recognizable purpose or point of home visits might actually be" (Heritage & Sefi, 1992, pp. 412–413). To resolve this dilemma, in the absence of mother-initiated requests for advice, HVs may attempt to unearth a problem through focused questioning, or through proposing a hypothetical problem "and then offering advice on it" (p. 385).

Conceivably, the oncologists in the current study could skip phase 2 discussions and simply prescribe an adjuvant therapy treatment regimen to the patient, sending her home with instructions on where and when to appear for treatment if she so chooses, once side effects and risk have been discussed. However, no oncologist in this data ever does that. Instead, they begin most visits by asking the patient to discuss her situation and concerns. Thus, the doctors in this study work to gain entry to their job of informing and recommending by soliciting patient perspectives and then proposing to address them during the visit. They may or may not actually address each concern raised.

This activity at the outset of the clinic visit, initiated by the oncologist, apparently works to get the patient to request advice. This action (of requesting advice) establishes the relevance of subsequent advice-giving in three respects (Heritage & Sefi, 1992, p. 370): (1) it establishes the problem area, (2) it establishes the requester's uncertainty about that area, and (3) it establishes alignment of the asker as a prospective recipient of advice, legitimizing the subsequent delivery of advice. In effect, by asking for the patient's perspective on her condition, the doctor gains entry into and legitimizes his or her role as advice-giver. Though we might imagine that doctors do not need legitimizing in the eyes of patients, it is evident from these data that these oncologists do go through such a conversational routine to establish the relevance of their role as advice-giver on this particular occasion.

The following excerpts are examples of how the oncologist elicits the patient's reason for the visit. Notice that just prior to, or close on the heels of, that elicitation, they may refer to having read the patient's record. Given that these oncologists already know most of what is needed to treat the patient, the question is raised, "What is this elicitation accomplishing?" or, "What is it doing at this point?" I am proposing that this solves the ticket-of-entry problem for the physician. We see that, later in the encounter, the oncologist either reiterates some aspect of what the patient has disclosed or supplies certain details that the patient may have left out. This is a notable pattern in much of the data. The information elicited in these early moments is frequently referred to later in the talk, making the elicitation functional in terms of arguments for treatment to be made later in phase 5.

Excerpt 5a

DR 8	A→	What's your understanding of (.) why
		Doctor H referred you.
PT 46		Hopefully for treatment. *Or the decision
		as to treatment*=
DR 8		=(For/your) decision as to the treatment)=
PT 46		=right.
DR 8	B→	Okay. Now what's your understanding o:::f (0.5)
PT 46		((clears throat))
DR 8		of where you stand at this point. In terms
		of (your breast).
		(1.5)
PT 46		where I stand.
DR 8		Yeah.
		(1.0)
PT 46		I::: (1.5) I don't know if I've even
		attempted to put it into (.) thoughts or
		words.
		(2.5)
		I::: (4.0) *I::::* (2.0) I know that
		it's not the simplest,. I don't believe it
		(.)
		I believe that uh::: (2.0) if (.) the lymph
		nodes were not invo::lved uh:: ((unintelligble
		due to microphone noise and noise in hallway))
DR 8		Okay. Uhm? Now. (1.0) In Doctor H's notes, uh and
		some a the
		other records that came, there was s- some

Excerpt 6a

63	DR 2	A→	Good. All right. Now, what was your understanding as
64			far as what Doctor [L] told ya about the tumor and
65			what it invo::lved and, things like that. Let's work
66			from there what what you know so far=
67	PT 2		=Ya mean what's gonna happen now?
68	DR 2	B→	Or where exactly the tumor was n how far it was
69			invo::lved and and what possibilities are (there)
70			for further therapy.
71	PT 2		Well the only thing I know is I had big lump here
72	DR 2		mm
73	PT 2		and they took the breast off they took, fifteen
74			laydaments or whatever you call em out from under my
75			arm,
76	DR 2		Lymph nodes. Right=
77	PT 2		=okay=
78	DR 2		=okay
79	PT 2		And thirteen of em was clear and two was cancer.
80	DR 2		Aright so that's exactly my understanding too.

The first two arrows (A and B) in each of these excerpts mark where the physician elicits, through an initial question and further reformulation of the question, the patient's orientation to her visit that day—"where she stands after surgery." In excerpt 5a, at line 25, the doctor refers to having read the notes on the patient's case. In excerpt 6a, about a minute prior to the talk reproduced here, the doctor explicitly stated that he had read the patient's record; at line 80 of excerpt 6a, he now indicates that his and the patient's understanding of her condition are in alignment. The doctor has succeeded in getting a formulation of the problem (positive lymph nodes) from the patient and in this way advice-giving becomes relevant as the next two excerpts show.

Excerpts 5b and 6b are continuations of the two previous excerpts. Here the doctor returns to the patient's original description of her medical condition to focus on the information about positive lymph nodes. This leads to an account, by the doctor, of why the patient is being referred for additional treatment. As we see in chapter 5, the positive lymph nodes serve as the cornerstone of the doctors' recommendations in phase 5.

Excerpt 5b (continuation of 5a)

140	DR 8	Okay. Let me make sure I've got everything
141		straight from your records. You had an
142		abnormal mammogram,
143	PT 46	Yes.
144	DR 8	You ha::::d s uh simple mastectomy initially
145	PT 46	[mm
146		[on both sides. The:: one on the left (.) wa
147		they were concerned about it so they went
148		back an (.) did a more extensive operation,
149	PT 46	mm
150	DR 8	and took some lymph nodes out.
151	PT 46	Yes.
152	DR 8	An:: [:d
153		loudspeaker [( ) line nine oh
154	DR 8	those lymph nodes were positive.
155	PT 46	eh
156	DR 8	That's (.) why (.) they're referring you
157		here.
158	PT 46	Yeah.

Excerpt 6b (continuation of 6a)

119	DR 2	Okay. Well, what I thought we'd do- I'd
120		examine you and then we'd talk a bit about
121		what it means to have a couple of lymph
122		nodes positive in breast cancer [. . .]

In both of these cases, and others not shown (*n* = 5), the oncologist's uptake of the patient's description of her condition focuses on the patient's lymph node status (at lines 150–156 of excerpt 5b and lines 121–122 of excerpt 6b). This becomes the basis of the recommendation to further treat the patient with adjuvant chemotherapy. When the lymph node information is not brought out by the doctor's general elicitation of the patient's understanding of her condition, the doctor brings it up as a rhetorical request, "Let me make sure I've got everything straight . . ." (lines 140–141, excerpt 5b).

The initial sequences (excerpts 5a and 6a) and their continuations (5b and 6b) are analogous to what Maynard (1991b, 1992) has identified as a "perspective-display" sequence, a conversational move initiated by a clinician to set up a "hospitable environment" for delivery of information (Maynard, 1992, p. 336). By asking the patient to disclose her reason for being at the doctor's office, the doctor not only sets up the interactional framework (establishing a ticket of entry to advice-giving) but also implicates the patient in the delivery of the news to come about possible need for further treatment. The doctor can use the patient's reporting of her positive lymph nodes later in phase 5 to launch into a discussion of the mechanics of cancer, available treatments and their side effects.

In summary, phase 2 is characterized by the doctor's elicitation of the patient's understanding of her current medical condition. He may elicit both the events leading up to the diagnosis and the patient's perspective on the purpose of her visit. Then, the doctor's questions are formulated so that the patient is directed to discuss her situation "since the surgery." This tends to bring out questions that the patient has, and also works to elicit the patient's knowledge of lymph node involvement. In this way, lymph node involvement is brought into focus.

The elicitation activity of phase 2 is a conversational sequence that works to license the physician's dispensing of his or her duties. This is evidenced by the patient's response with a request for advice and information. The opening sequence appears to provide the physician with a ticket of entry into the task of informing patients and making recommendations. The formulation of the elicitation activity, which is quite similar to Maynard's perspective-display sequence, involves the patient in the delivery of the news to come that further treatment may be needed.

The allocation of turns in phase 2 is activated by the doctor at the outset. The physician initiates the encounter, asking the patient to recount her understanding of her condition. Patients take extended turns in this phase in which they tell the story of their illness and also raise their concerns, asking questions of the doctor. In phase 3, discussed in section 3.5, turn types change considerably: The doctor asks specific medical and demographic questions and the patient provides short answers. Before going to phase 3, however, readers should take note of the transition from phase 2 to phase 3.

3.4 *Transition from Phase 2 to Phase 3*

This section looks briefly at the transition from phase 2 to phase 3. These transitions further exemplify the doctor's orientation to these encounters as agenda-based.

Excerpt 7 illustrates an elicitation of concerns (phase 2 activity) followed by a topic shift into medical and demographic information (phase 3 activity). The doctor moves within a single turn from one phase to the next.

Excerpt 7

18	DR 7	→	Why don't you start by letting me know why
19			ya- why you're here.
20	PT 53		O [kay::
21	DR 7	→	[what I can do for you.
22	PT 53		Well the last I had seen Doctor A uh:: he didn't
23			think that I needed any (.) treatment. But he
24			wanted to discuss it with you.
25	DR 7		Uh huh.
26	PT 53		And uhm I just wanted to find out a little more
27			about the (.) the- I guess it's the <u>adj</u>uvant
28			chemo [therapy
29	DR 7		[Right.
30	PT 53		that we're gonna discuss.
31	DR 7		Right.
32	PT 53		And just find out (.) whether we ( ) really do
33			it or not.
34	DR 7	→	Right. Right. You're twenty-two?

Here, at the outset of this visit, the doctor invites the patient to disclose her reason for being at the office, even though he has already spoken to Doctor A and has a "head start" in reading the record (lines 5–7, data not shown). At the arrows at lines 18 and 21, evidence indicates that the doctor explicitly invites the patient to provide her perspective, despite his prior knowledge of her case. As mentioned, this is a phase 2 activity, clearly establishing the purpose of the visit and placing the patient in the recipient of advice position. The doctor provides receipt tokens ("right." at lines 29, 31, 34) indicating no current objection to the patient's formulation of the reason for her visit; that is the doctor displays some degree of agreement on the purpose of the visit by passing "the opportunity to take a turn" (Schegloff, 1982). At the last line (34), the doctor bridges the two phases by first receipting the patient's talk then shifting to medical history, within his own turn, by asking the question, "You're twenty-two?" This turn marks the beginning of the gathering of the patient's medical history. This question does not refer to preceding talk but projects forward to a new topic. In this way the doctor closes the phase 2 elicitation of patient perspective on the problem and has moved the agenda into phase 3 where pointed questions are asked and the patient supplies short answers—very short in comparison to phase 2—as discussed next in section 3.5.

3.5 *Medical History Gathering in Phase 3*

The gathering of medical history, the predominant activity of phase 3, has been described extensively elsewhere (Byrne & Long, 1976; Mishler, 1984). Therefore, I discuss this aspect of the adjuvant therapy discussion only briefly. Essentially, during this phase the oncologists ask questions that elicit short answers or yes/no responses concerning medical and demographic facts not related to the patient's cancer. At this point questions are asked about usual medications, other surgeries, family situation, employment status, and so on. The doctors rarely do any reformulating or clarifying of their questions.

During this phase, patients provide one-word or short sentence responses; often the doctor's question elicits a simple yes/no response. In this way, the allocation of turn types is distinctly different from phase 2, in which patients take extended turns and doctor questions can be rather general (e.g., "what's your understanding of where you stand," as in excerpt 5a). And the doctors' questions in phase 2 are often reformulated in response to patient requests for clarification (as in excerpt 6a).

In contrast, excerpt 8 is clearly marked as medical history taking. The doctor poses questions which elicit specific medical information, and the patient responds with little elaboration—unless requested to do so by the doctor.

Excerpt 8

DR 5 Okay. Do you have any history of any heart trouble.
PT 28 No.
DR 5 Okay. Have you ever had hepatitis or yellow jaundice.
PT 28 No.
DR 5 Okay. No kidney trouble that you're aware of.
PT 28 Nnnnot what uh well I had kidney infection here in fact in uh, before
DR 5 Just before you came in, that's right.
PT 28 Um-hum.
DR 5 Okay, but that cleared up (.) with
PT 28 Oh [yeah.

89	DR 5	[antibiotics and [so forth.
90	PT 28	[Yeah. Right.
91	DR 5	Okay.
92		(3.0)
93		Are you treated for high blood pressure at all.
94	PT 28	I have blood pressure pills.
95		(2.0)
96	DR 5	What's what what medicine, what what do you take for
97		that. You know the name of it?
98	PT 28	Day HY, I don't know.
99	DR 5	HCTZ.=
100	PT 28	=Could be, um-hum.
101	DR 5	Hydrocortithiazol. Twenty-five or fifty.
102	PT 28	Twenty-five.
103	DR 5	Twenty-five. One or two a day.
104	PT 28	One.
105		(4.0)
106	PT 28	(sniffs)
107	DR 5	And the diabetes you've had for about five years?
108	PT 28	Um-hum.
109		(4.0)
110	DR 5	Has the diabetes affected your eyesight at all?
111	PT 28	No.
112	DR 5	Okay.=
113	PT 28	=I keep a close watch on my eyes.
114	DR 5	Good. Good.
115		(2.5)

After each "okay" utterance there is final, falling intonation and, as defined by Sacks et al. (1974), there is also syntactic completion (lines 78, 80, 82). In other words, there is a completeness to the utterance. Here, the final, falling intonation can indicate a place for speaker transition (a transition relevance place), and, as illustrated in the next excerpt, patients do sometimes step in to take the floor after a doctor utters an "Okay." In this excerpt, however, the patient continues to pass the floor back to the doctor by choosing not speak after his "Okay" receipt tokens. She clearly orients to this as a question and answer sequence—a "history taking," one with which we are all familiar from visiting doctors' offices.

Note that she also does not step in to take a turn at the long pauses after lines 92, 95, and 105; the doctor initiates the adjacency pairs. Nearly all the patient's responses are short, factual, and unelaborated. This represents typical turn types and typical allocation of turns within standard medical interviews.

The next excerpt shows a disruption of phase 3 by a patient who does not stay within the confines of the medical history taking format. The participants are in the midst of phase 3 when a slight foray into troubles-telling is initiated by the patient. This excerpt, and the notion of troubles-telling, is taken up in further detail in section 3.6; for the time being excerpt 9 takes a cursory look at troubles-telling in terms of how the doctor maintains his footing within a phase 3 activity.

Excerpt 9

126	DR 2	Any other surgeries or anything?
127	PT 2	N::aw I had um (0.5) hysterectomy in seventy.
128		[I dunno-
129	DR 2	[What was the reason for that.
130	PT 2	Well I was pregnant, (0.5) and I didn't want no more,
131		so they took the uh baby and uh had the hysterectomy
132		when I (had that one).
133	DR 2	*Okay.*
134	PT 2	And then I had appendicitis.
135		(1.3)
136	PT 2	*That was a nightmare*
137	DR 2	Okay. AND any other medical problems like high
138		blood pressure, diabe:tes, heart trouble,=kidney
139		trouble,
140	PT 2	[m
141	DR 2	[anything like that?
142	PT 2	No, I'm a healthy specimen.
143	DR 2	Nk. All right. You're (.) uh::m an East [city name]
144		resident here?
145	PT 2	[mm
146	DR 2	[You live here? You lived here most a your life?
147	PT 2	All my life.
148	DR 2	*All your life. Okay.* And uh
149	PT 2	((sniffs))
150	DR 2	are you married, single, divorced?
151	PT 2	Married, Have six children and seven grandchildren.

The excerpt begins with the doctor asking about "other" surgeries as part of his gathering of medical information. The patient mentions a hysterectomy, and as she begins to (possibly) elaborate in some way, the doctor also begins speaking (lines 128 and 129). This overlap may indicate the doctor's orientation to the patient's turn as being complete after the simple report of having had the surgery in 1970. He treats her turn as complete at this point and his request for elaboration gains the floor (line 129). Following the doctor's receipt token ("Okay.") in line 133, the patient then mentions she had appendicitis (line 134). Mentioning appendicitis implies appendectomy, a legitimate response to his surgery question. But she then comments on that as a nightmarish experience. The doctor merely receipts this turn but does not respond further. He pursues his line of questioning relative to any other "medical problems." The rest of his questions are focused to elicit facts from the patient (patient's place and duration of residence, marital status) and he receives focused, one-word, or short-phrase answers.

Both of the preceding excerpts, drawn from phase 3, are easily recognizable as medical history gathering, and it is worth noting how the turn types and allocation of turns differ from those in phase 2. Turns here are shorter, the responses by patients more concise, and the questions by doctors more focused on medical facts. Within phase 3, the doctor manages the talk with little resistance from the patient. Indeed, patients easily pass the floor to the doctor with few exceptions. Excerpt 9 demonstrated the doctor's avoidance of the topic of the patient's "nightmarish" appendicitis, by choosing to keep the talk within the confines of phase 3 topics. I now turn to this phenomenon in some detail to complete this chapter's discussion of the organization of talk in the adjuvant therapy encounter and the ways in which information is managed by the oncologists in this institutional setting.

3.6 Resistance to Troubles-Telling: Orientation to a Service Encounter

As noted thus far, these oncology visits are organized as task- or agenda-based interactions in which the physician invokes a preferred order of events to manage the release of information. This agenda-based organization is one aspect of how these oncology visits are constructed as institutional service encounters. Service encounters, whether institutional or in ordinary conversation, are defined by Jefferson and Lee (1992) as those in which the focal object is a problem and its properties; the upshot of this focusing is often advice-giving. In contrast, in conversations in which one speaker's experiences are presented as difficulties or "troubles," advice need not be the upshot and can in fact cause disruption in the talk.

In the data presented for the current study, there are moments when events mentioned by patients are attended to by the physicians and other times when they are not. Discussion of personal difficulties that arise outside the context of the cancer itself or the cancer treatment are generally resisted. This is apparent in moments when a troubles-worthy event is mentioned, but there is lack of uptake by the physician and lack of subsequent pursuance by the patient. Such events range from patient reports of their children's drug problems to reports of a tooth being knocked out during the anesthesia procedure. It is important to note that when the oncologist "resists" engaging as troubles-recipient (i.e., does not offer solace or commiseration), patients rarely pursue the topic. In this way the absence of elaboration of personal troubles can be seen as cooperatively maintained by the doctor and the patient. Only when the trouble relates to the cancer itself or the proposed treatment do the oncologists take a more troubles-accepting stance. Resistance to troubles-telling can be demonstrated by looking at a few contrasting cases.

Excerpt 10 is a portion of excerpt 9, just discussed in the context of describing phase 3 activities. The longer excerpt was part of an unfolding question-answer sequence in which the doctor is collecting relevant medical history. Here, we focus on how the doctor maintains a service encounter orientation (identification of problems and their properties) in the face of the patient's attempt to introduce her troubles into the talk. Prior to what is given in this excerpt, the doctor had asked the patient about "any other surgeries" to which she replied by describing her hysterectomy. That is the talk that the doctor receipts at line 133 ("Okay"):

Excerpt 10

133	DR 2	Okay.
134	PT 2	And then I had appendicitis.
135		(1.3)
136	PT 2	*That was a nightmare*
137	DR 2	Okay. AND any other medical problems like high
138		blood pressure, diabe:tes, heart trouble,=kidney
139		trouble,

The patient continues (line 134) after the receipt token not by naming another surgery, a possible contribution at this point, but by invoking a situation that might demand surgery (appendicitis). Following the pause in line 135, the patient continues with an assessment of her appendicitis, "that was a nightmare," uttered at reduced volume. This is a move distinctly different from her contributions thus far in the talk. Up to this point the patient had been providing factual answers regarding her medical history and general state of health. There is no uptake of the patient's assessment. Rather than take up this indication of troubles (patient's nightmarish appendicitis) as a discussable topic, the doctor receipts her remark with an "okay" but continues with a new question. He links to his prior agenda with the conjunction "and" uttered at increased volume relative to the surrounding talk (line 137).

Prefacing a next question by "and" introduces the question as a continuation of prior talk (Heritage & Sorjonen, 1994; Schiffrin, 1987). Thus, the patient's remark is treated as irrelevant to the ongoing activity of asking questions and getting answers—a distinctly service-oriented stance. In this sequential context immediately following the indication of the troublesworthy nightmarish experience, the doctor's contribution may be viewed as a part of an array of *troubles-telling exit devices* (see Jefferson, 1984a, pp. 192–194). Such conversational moves are "topically disjunctive" in that whatever comes next does not emerge from nor is it topically coherent with the troubles mentioned (Jefferson, 1984a, p. 194). The doctor does not affiliate in any way with the patient and her experience but moves away from any talk of her nightmarish appendicitis, continuing his collection of medical facts from her. With this same patient, later during the medical history gathering, the doctor also passes the opportunity to make relevant topics such as the patient's children smoking crack and the patient's own relinquishing a habit of heavy drinking (data not shown). These may be topics pursued in some other types of medical encounters, and certainly in a more troubles-receptive atmosphere, but during these visits the doctor receipts them in a manner similar to the troubles-exiting noted earlier.

Excerpt 11 provides another example of how doctors in this data do not quickly engage in commiserating with their patients. In excerpt 11, Patient 27 reiterates that the news that she might now need chemotherapy (when originally told that she would not) has come as "quite a shock." She uses the phrase "quite a shock" twice in her extended turn—a turn punctuated by three long pauses and repeated reformulations of her dismay over learning that she would, after all, require chemotherapy. Her extended turn can be analyzed as being in pursuit of a response by the doctor, which she does not receive until line 89. Finally, at the end of this extended turn, the doctor acknowledges Patient 27's distress after a 6-second pause.

Excerpt 11

68	PT 27	and then it- I mean came to (.) quite a shock when
69		I- mean I had my uhh (decisions) and he asked me
70		to see Doctor S, you know that uh (.) about what he
71		was gonna say, and uh (.) I mean I was a little
72		prepared for it but not (.) not really. An it came as
73		quite a shock=I mean ( ) an especially when he (.)
74		he says it's a really (.) strong chemotherapy.
75		(2.0)
76		I was just wondering whether that was necessary.
77		(2.0)
78		Under the circumstances if the (thought)- ya know
79		since (.) only one lymph node was involved.
80		(6.0)
81		But I did really feel like ya know after the uhm (.)
82		the operation and the (.) X-ray treatment that that
83		would, that was gonna be it. And I assumed they
84		would (.) ya know keep track of me:, and have me
85		come for regular check ups and that kind of thing
86		but (.) I thought basically the the worst part was
87		over.
88		(6.0)
89	DR 4	Right. This knocks you off your pins.
90	PT 27	Really.
91		(2.0)
92	PT 27	*This is such a shock*
93		(3.5)
94	DR 4	Any other questions or things you want
95		(1.5)
96		me to help you with here today?

The doctor provides one comment which takes up the patient's distress over the unexpected news that she will need chemotherapy. He commiserates with her by agreeing that such a course of events can be unsettling. The patient reiterates her sense of "shock" at line 92 but receives no further comment from the doctor. Rather, he reintroduces the activity of gathering patient concerns to be addressed (lines 94–96).

The final excerpt is the only one in which a doctor does any extended receipt of troubles-talk by a patient. This is taken from the most contentious of the visits in the data. Throughout the encounter the patient has been speaking very pessimistically; she is concerned that she may start treatment and when it is shown to be ineffective that the doctors will abandon her. She has been referring to a woman in the waiting room who is now facing a cancer recurrence—she mentions that woman again at line 242, but it fails to get a response. The long pause at line 244, followed by the doctor's move to discuss the recommendation, clearly shows some disruption in the talk. The doctor relinquishes his troubles-receptive stance and attempts to move forward to the topic of the recommendation.

Excerpt 12

202	PT 37		(All I need to hear) on this (.) field
203			I'll tell you.
204	DR 4		We give-
205	PT 37		Sickening really.
206	DR 4	→	*yeah. [It's disappointing.*
207	PT 37		[I mean it doesn't bother you
208			until you get it. But uh (.) all this
209			research and everything. What are they
210			doin just spending all the money? and
211			not coming up with nothin. It's just
212			ridiculous.
213			(1.0)
214			Millions and millions a dollars (.)
215			spent on something and they sstill don't
216			have a cure.
217	DR 4	→	*That's right. That's a tough problem.*
218			(1.0)
219	PT 37		I mean I can understand now why people
220			would just (.) not even have a breast
221			removed. I felt better before I had my
222			breast removed than I feel now.
223	DR 4	→	mm.
224	PT 37		It's been hell.
			.
			.
			.
241			(2.5)

PT 37	She was a good example of what uh I can
	expect.
	(4.5)
DR 4	What we are currently recommending, uh:m
	for patients in your situation, with (.)
	more than ten lymph nodes involved, is
	(.) a study that we're doin.

In this excerpt, the doctor takes two turns to provide supporting remarks (at lines 206 and 217) to the patient. Both are formulations that revise the patient's assessments: she says "sickening" he echoes with "disappointing" she says "ridiculous" he forms his remark with "tough problem." Though his reformulated remarks are less strong, they still take up the patient's apparent complaints about the system and about her own condition. The doctor also passes the floor back to the patient (line 223) giving her the opportunity to continue her expression of disappointment. These passing moves and displays of commiseration allow the patient to express her unhappiness and frustration; however, this behavior by the doctor comes only after the patient has shown considerable resistance to the doctor's contributions thus far. Apparently, it takes considerable pursuance by the patient to get even the minimal alignment with her troubles that is evident from Doctor 4 in this excerpt.

3.7 Conclusion

In this chapter I have outlined the four central phases of the oncology visit and treated the first two phases in detail. The import of phase 4, the physical examination (though not audio-recorded) is discussed in chapter 4. And phase 5 of the visit (the recommendation), is examined in detail in chapter 5.

The analysis presented in this chapter reveals how clinic visits to discuss adjuvant therapy are constructed as agenda-based encounters in which doctors work to proceed through a sequence of activities. This was demonstrated by looking at the doctor's explicit references to the activities to be accomplished, as well as the doctor's management of the talk by delaying certain topics. Finally, this chapter noted how the doctor's resistance to troubles-telling further underscores these visits as service encounters, occasions for giving and receiving information as opposed to commiserating with the patient.

Management of the agenda in the ways outlined provides a new perspective on how it is that asymmetrical control of medical encounters is achieved. The shape of the turns—extended patient turns in phase 2 as opposed to briefer (even minimal yes/no) responses in phase 3—contributes to the marking off of topical phases within the encounter. And although this is common to medical visits, it was noted that patients are allowed uninterrupted turns in phase 2, which is in sharp contrast to findings from investigations of general medical visits. Further, the dispreference for patient questions—a topic to be taken up further in chapter 4—may be related to the sequential placement of the patient's question, that is, the phase of the agenda in which they are placed (see also ten Have, 1991). This refines our understanding of the recurrent observation that patient questions are dispreferred in medical settings (Frankel, 1989; West, 1983; West & Frankel, 1991).

The elicitation of the patient's questions, concerns, and understanding of her current situation works to license the physician to proceed to the activity of providing information and making a recommendation. Gaining such a ticket of entry was first discussed as a phenomenon occurring in ordinary talk (Sacks, 1972) and has been evaluated in one other institutional setting (Heritage & Sefi, 1992). This concept, if extended to more areas of talk-in-interaction, could prove fruitful for understanding in a more detailed and orderly way how people enter cooperatively into a wide range of activities.

These observations combine to give a sense of how it is that oncologists and their patients with breast cancer move through a set of activities that contributes to the overall sense that they are working together toward the rather serious activity of discussing adjuvant therapy. Breast cancer can be life threatening, and oncologists need the patient's cooperation to help save the patient's life. As such, these encounters are structured from the outset as professional, institutional visits in which expertise and knowledge will be shared—but only at the appropriate time. The "appropriateness" of the timing of their discussion of adjuvant therapy is not, I believe, just for the sake of orderliness. It is constitutive of the role that the oncologist has as gatekeeper and as such instantiates his or her expertise in the setting. In the next chapter, we further explore this question of expertise as well as the patient's role as an educable novice.

4

Discourse Identities: Establishing Participant Roles as Doctor and Patient

The previous chapter examined the ways in which the adjuvant therapy consultation is structured as a service encounter, as a legitimate occasion for giving and receiving advice or recommendations. Specifically, I noted the major activity phases of the encounter, the characteristic allocation of turns and turn types within phases, and the doctor's orientation to an agenda for the visit. Both topic control and resistance to patient troubles-talk were notable mechanisms for maintaining the service orientation of the visit. Importantly, the doctor elicits the patient's concerns about, and understanding of, her condition, which works to cast her provisionally in the role of advice seeker and co-implicates her in the recommendation to come.

The significance of these observations relates to the general goal of identifying patterns of action and of talk—observable facts—that constitute the adjuvant therapy discussion. Having laid the foundation in this way, the current chapter further examines what contributes to the accomplishment of these visits as legitimate occasions for giving recommendations. A central concern of this investigation is to understand how expertise is instantiated in the often unnoticed details of talk-in-interaction. This question is of great interest in-as-much as it helps to understand why one person might cooperate in receiving advice from another. One participant, in the provisional role of advice-giver, must be treated as expert in some way. This is key for understanding how it is that patients may be persuaded to take a particular course of action.

I propose that service providers must display appropriate knowledge and expertise to make relevant their service or advice and have that knowledgeability accepted by the recipient through interaction. The potential recipient of the service must present herself as someone in need of the advice or service being offered. In the current data, breast cancer patients are meeting with a person who, according to some third party, has expertise in the area of concern to them. Generally, these patients have been referred by another physician. Despite the fact that the oncology clinic visit is one in which the patient "knows" that she will be meeting a specialist, and the doctor knows that he or she will be meeting a certain kind of patient, I will show that conversational work actually brings the identities of "doctor/expert" and "patient/novice" to the fore on a moment-to-moment basis. I work from the premise that doctors are not expert service providers simply because they carry specialized knowledge in their heads; doctors are experts by virtue of (1) the expertise/knowledge they display or invoke in the encounter and (2) the conversational moves they initiate which establish them as gatekeepers to knowledge. For their part, patients treat doctors as people with expertise by asking for help and guidance. The doctor's expertise is, therefore, not just a fact of his or her professional preparation but also a cooperatively constructed social phenomenon.

To explore these claims about the construction of discourse identities through conversation, I look first at one oncologist-patient encounter in detail. The single case provides a sequentially coherent view of how participant roles are managed as the interaction progresses toward the recommendation. After looking at the single case, I isolate one aspect of that encounter—patient appeals for information—and discuss that phenomenon by drawing on other cases from the data. Finally, this chapter looks briefly at how patients are constructed as educable people in these encounters.

4.1 A Single Case

In the 7 minutes that make up the phase 2 and 3 activities of the meeting between Doctor 2 and Patient 2, the two participants accomplish a great deal in terms of establishing who has access to what kinds of information. The display of knowledge is one mechanism by which members identify and locate roles within the myriad identities they could potentially invoke. In excerpt 13, the patient is being treated as someone who has access to knowledge about the time of the discovery of a palpable breast lump and her reason for delaying a breast biopsy.

This type of event has been termed a "B-event" by Labov and Fanshell (1977, pp. 62–64). It is some event to which the recipient of the talk/question has primary access, as opposed to an "AB-event," something to which both parties would have access (or an "A-event," something to which only the non-responder would have access). As Heritage and Roth assert, "An utterance [formulated as a B-event] makes a recipient's confirmation or denial relevant in the next turn" (Heritage & Roth, 1995, p. 10). In other words, asking about or assessing some event which only one party (the recipient) has knowledge of (a "B-event") makes verification, endorsement, or disavowal an appropriate next move by the recipient.

In excerpt 13, the discovery of the breast lump is investigated as a B-event by the doctor; he formulates this as information to which only the patient has access. Importantly, although the patient is treated as the authority on her health history, the assessment of her behavior as a patient is implicitly negative. At the outset of the encounter the patient is asked to review the story of the discovery of the lump in her breast and the apparent delay of the biopsy leading to the diagnosis. The patient accounts for the latter by saying that she had no insurance.

Excerpt 13

1	DR 2	An this was (.) a long time ago? er,
2	PT 2	mmm
3		(1.0)
4		No the first time I noticed it was back in
5		September * (I think.)*
6	DR 2	A:ndh, (0.6) what was the reasoning or what what
7		was thuh (.) the a (.) reason for the fact that (.)
8		took so long to get it (0.5) *biop [sied.*
9	PT 2	[Well when I first
10		found it I didn't have any insurance.
11	DR 2	*I see. Okay. [(well that's)*
12	PT 2	[And I- that'ss all I have to say
13		[hunh hunh hunh ((laugh))
14	DR 2	[I can understand that.
15	PT 2	[((sniffs))
16	DR 2	[Okay. So eventually you went and had a biopsy done,
17	PT 2	[mm?

18 DR 2 [and they found that it was a tumor or a
19 cancer?
20 (1.2)
21 Recommended a mastectomy.
22 PT 2 Right.
23 (1.0)

The doctor's initial question (line 1) presents a candidate answer embedded within his question (Pomerantz, 1988), though the "er" trail-off leaves the door open for the patient to offer an alternative. The candidate answer here is that the discovery of the lump happened "a long time ago." By hedging the formulation (with the "er" trail-off), the doctor's question introduces the potential relevance of some other answer to be offered by the patient. He works to leave the door open to a statement that the discovery of the breast lump did *not,* in fact, happen a long time ago. It is allowable here for the patient to offer an alternative to the doctor's characterization of the event. The patient's self-knowledge is treated as legitimate.

In lines 4 and 5, the patient directly negates the doctor's characterization of the event and elaborates that the discovery of the lump happened "back in September." By refuting that she found the lump "a long time ago" the patient diminishes the possibility that she may be viewed as careless. Ignoring a palpable breast lump could be viewed as negligent behavior.

The doctor continues his "line of questioning" with delays and hesitations. The topic to come (patient's delaying of biopsy) is delayed and hedged several times in lines 6–8. The doctor phrases his question with an assumption of reasonableness on the part of the patient ("what was the reasoning . . .") yet treats the delay of the biopsy as an "accountable" action, that is, one that deviates from some norm (Heritage, 1984, pp. 115–120). In this way, the doctor works to get the patient to provide him with information while treating her action as potentially sanctionable.

The patient's response at lines 9–10 is evidence that the doctor's request for an account is hearable as a negative assessment. The doctor's turn-in-progress (lines 6–8) projects a question that is treated by the patient as an implied criticism. As Atkinson and Drew (1979) have demonstrated, an accusation makes relevant a denial in the next slot. And in line 9, the patient precisely places the start of her talk in anticipation of the doctor's term "biopsy." Prefaced by "well," which is often produced as a preface to disagreement (Pomerantz, 1984), the patient stakes an early claim on the next turn, carefully placing her "well" to overlap the key word (biopsy) in the doctor's question. She thus leaves the account for her action ("I didn't have any insurance") in the clear. In this way, the patient quickly refutes the negative implication of the doctor's question and conveys "vigorous rejection of the suggested criticism" (Heritage & Roth, 1995, pp. 16–17).

Further, at line 11, the doctor accepts the patient's implied reason for the delay of the biopsy ("I see. Okay.") and begins to elaborate. The patient also starts speaking at the transition relevance place. She regains the floor with the conjunctive "And I-" projecting perhaps a further account of her possibly negligent behavior, though she cuts herself off and attempts to close the topic ("that's all I have to say") on line 12.[1] The doctor's statement, "I can understand that" (line 14), is hearable as an understanding of her account as both plausible and reasonable, as something he can accept.

The doctor then recaps the patient's biopsy/surgery story (lines 16–21) and invites the patient's confirmation of his report by his use of rising intonation at line 19. In this way, the doctor formulates as a B-event what could have been either their shared knowledge (an AB-event) or only the patient's knowledge (a B-event). In this way, he treats the patient as expert on her medical history. The patient ratifies his telling as being "right" in line 22. She moves thus, conversationally, to indicate that doctor and patient are in alignment in terms of the medical-historical facts.

The preceding analysis of the first 45 seconds of the consultation demonstrates a number of important points. First, the patient is treated as the authority on her health history; she is expected to know when she first found a palpable breast lump and what caused her to delay having it biopsied. Second, by asking the patient to account for her action of delaying the biopsy, the doctor treats her past behavior as problematic, thus presenting himself as someone in a position to judge her action. In fact, he offers an assessment of her reasoning (line 14), marking it as acceptable or understandable. Finally, the patient moves to ratify the doctor's synopsis of her recent medical history, casting herself in the position of expert on her health history, a person in the position to ratify another's telling of it. Conversationally, the two participants are brought into alignment over the recent facts. But this brief exchange of information, where the patient is in possession of facts, is soon reversed as the talk continues (as transcribed in excerpt 14).

Excerpt 14 is the immediate continuation of the previous talk. The doctor states that he has obtained and read the record of the patient's recent hospitalization. He then turns the talk to the topic of how the patient has been feeling.

Excerpt 14

24	DR 2	I have all the records from your hospitalizations=*I
25		have a good idea of what happened after that.*
26		How've ya been feelin?
27		(0.8)
28	PT 2	I feel (0.5) pretty good. But I'm frustrated . . .

The doctor clearly and unproblematically invokes his access to the patient's confidential medical records. The patient presents no objection to this fact. By citing his access to the patient's records and to knowledge about the events following the biopsy, the doctor openly displays his institutional authority. Friends, for example, do not usually arm themselves with medical records for a discussion of "how've ya been feelin?" The roles of institutional representative and service seeker are brought clearly into focus at this moment.

As their discussion continues (excerpt 15), the patient reports that she's "tired" all the time and does not know how long she is going to feel "that way." She asks the doctor if he is going to tell her. Thus she formulates the state of her personal well-being as information to which only the doctor has access. Curiously, then, the patient's well-being is formulated *by her* as a B-event in the doctor's domain.

Excerpt 15

28	PT 2	I feel (0.5) pretty good. But I'm frustrated as
29		hell cause I can't do nothin.
30		(0.8)
31		I'm tired all the time. N I walked up Monument
32		Street yesterday, pay the gas n electric bill n come
33		home, I died the rest a the day. It took all my
34		strength to do that.
35	DR 2	mm
36	PT 2	An I don't know how long I'm gonna feel that
37		way.=You gonna tell me?
38	DR 2	Well how long ya been home altogether.
39	PT 2	hhhhhh ((sigh)) I think I got out the seventeenth.
40		(1.4)

The patient indicates her belief that the doctor knows something about her state of being that she herself does not know; specifically, how long she will be feeling poorly (lines 36–37). The patient presents herself as uncertain about her recent condition ("I don't know how long I'm gonna feel that way") whereas just moments before she easily offered an account regarding her delay of the biopsy. Now she proposes that she has a question about her physical and mental state that she cannot answer for herself. The patient treats the doctor as someone with expertise regarding her internal mental/physical state. The patient's question proposes that the doctor may be able to predict the duration of the feeling of fatigue she is experiencing. This question situates the doctor as one who is able to provide answers to questions that are not answerable by the patient herself.

Worth noting here is how content and format combine to underscore the doctor's position as the one in charge. The patient's question in lines 36–37 (How long will I feel this way?) is responded to by Doctor 2 with a question. In this way he moves into an interrogative sequence (Zimmerman, 1984, 1992). In a rather different institutional setting (i.e., calls for emergency assistance) such sequences move the caller's request for help forward; information crucial for dispatching assistance is elicited through the focused questions. In the current data it appears that an interrogative series is initiated by the doctor, though a response to the patient's question about fatigue is never actually answered. Instead, the doctor and patient move through a series of questions which culminate in the information that, in terms of the healing of the surgical site, everything is normal. The initiation of the interrogative sequence by the doctor maintains the turn format as an elicitation/response episode. Though he is the one "seeking information" as the questioner, the very fact of resisting her question (by not supplying an answer but initiating the interrogative series) casts him as the one in control of the trajectory of the talk at this point.

So in terms of the content of their interchange, the patient treats the doctor as someone who may be able to speak to her concerns about fatigue. In terms of the shape of the turns, the doctor enforces the turn format so that he is in the position of interrogator. Thus, the doctor's role as "expert in charge" is made manifest in both the content and the shape of their talk.

The following two excerpts further illustrate how these participants display and invoke knowledge and practices to situate themselves and the other in relevant roles of doctor/expert and patient/novice. This ongoing activity is integral to establishing the relative expertise of the participants, constructing the situation as one in which one person can help the other.

In excerpt 16, the interrogative series continues from excerpt 15 (though a few lines have been deleted here). The patient answers the doctor's new question about pain under the arm and then about the healing of her surgical site.

Excerpt 16

48 DR 2 Ya havin any pain?
49 PT 2 Just under my arm.
50 DR 2 ss-
51 PT 2 <u>None</u> up in here. Just under here.
52 DR 2 *Okay.* How'd the <u>heal</u>ing go with this *eh (.) the incision.*
53 PT 2 Uh::m Doctor[L] said it looks real good.
54 DR 2 *Okay.* When did you <u>see</u> him.
55 PT 2 Uh:: last week.

The patient provides a description of her pain in lines 49 and 51. She is once again the authority on her experience. Then, at line 53 she cites Doctor L as the source of the information about her healing process. The patient can relate her experience of pain, but when it comes to commenting on her healing, she treats that as answerable by an outside medical source (Doctor L). By establishing the state of her healing with reference to Doctor L, the patient categorizes that information as someone else's expert assessment.

This type of third-party reference has been analyzed as a conversational move which can be used to maintain neutrality (Clayman, 1988, 1992). Invoking a third party as a source of information shifts the burden of authorship away from the speaker. The patient thus does not present herself as the source of the assessment of her healing. She displays an orientation (line 53) to the dichotomy between expert/nonexpert with regard to her health, by proposing that it is Doctor L, not herself, who can assess her healing.

In excerpt 16, then, the "healing process" is being presented by the patient as a situation that is better assessed by another expert (Doctor L) than by the patient herself. Though these third-party references have been shown to mark conversational elements as possibly requiring "special handling" in news interviews (Clayman, 1992, p. 170), in excerpt 16 the doctor does not treat the patient's comment as in any way problematic or delicate. He does not, for example, ask, "But what do <u>you</u> think about the healing?" The reference to Doctor L's assessment is implicitly accepted as valid by Doctor 2 and he continues gathering information from the patient.

After Doctor 2 and Patient 2 finish the series of questions regarding the patient's surgical site, the doctor proceeds to elicit the patient's understanding of her condition.

Excerpt 17

63	DR 2	Good. All right. Now, what was your understanding as
64		far as what Doctor [L] told ya about the tumor and
65		what it invo::lved and, things like that. Let's work
66		from there what what you know so far=
67	PT 2	=Ya mean what's gonna happen now?
68	DR 2	Or where exactly the tumor was n how far it was
69		invo::lved and and what possibilities are (there)
70		for further therapy.
71	PT 2	Well the only thing I know is I had big lump here
72	DR 2	mm
73	PT 2	and they took the breast off they took, fifteen
74		laydaments or whatever you call em out from under my
75		arm,
76	DR 2	Lymph nodes. Right=
77	PT 2	=okay=
78	DR 2	=okay
79	PT 2	And thirteen of em was clear and two was cancer.
80	DR 2	Aright so that's exactly my understanding too.
81	PT 2	mm

In this stretch of talk, the doctor starts by wanting to know what the patient knows about her tumor. Doctor 2 invokes Doctor L as the primary source of the patient's information (line 64). In this way, he introduces a topic (outcome of surgery) for which he is proposing that the patient is not the expert on herself but is simply the reporter of others' assessments. By inviting the patient to frame her remarks in terms of what her other doctor said, the current doctor's mention of the third party works as an invitation for the patient to *not* be the principal responsible for her remarks, that is, to not be viewed as the expert on herself.

Indeed, when the patient answers the doctor's question she presents herself as "ignorant" or only minimally informed. At line 71 she prefaces her report by saying that the "only" thing she knows is that her breast was removed, that they evaluated her lymph nodes, and that two were cancerous. At line 74 the patient references her own possible mispronunciation of lymph nodes as "laydaments" by saying "whatever you call em." And, in fact, this elicits a correction by the doctor ("Lymph nodes. Right.") at line 76. In this moment, the patient presents herself as a novice in this arena and casts the doctor as the expert, orienting to him as a person able to know the proper term. At line 80, the doctor is now in the position of ratifying the patient's account, moving to treat this bit of knowledge as shared and displaying that their understandings are in alignment with one another (see also excerpt 13). These brief moments of shared understanding may work to establish a sense of rapport between the participants. So, although troubles-telling may not be an area in which doctors align with patients (see chapter 3, section 3.6), medical-historical facts are opportunities to share some knowledge or a viewpoint.

One final excerpt from this encounter provides further evidence of how doctor-patient roles are foregrounded in the talk. First, undergoing a physical exam (which occurs in 66% of the visits) is a nontrivial aspect of establishing doctor-patient roles and responsibilities. We do not usually let strangers examine our bodies in detail. The patient's agreement to submit to the examination ratifies her co-participant (i.e., the doctor) as someone with the institutional rights to perform such an activity.

Excerpt 18

231	DR 2	well what I thought we'd do is a
232	PT 2	((sniff))
233	DR 2	I'd examine you and the::n we'd talk a bit about (.)
234		what it means to have a couple of lymph nodes
235		positive (.) in breast cancer what we know about
236		that (.) an::d what it means (.) in t- in terms of
237		lon::g term outlook? (.) an::d (.) what kind of
238		treatments (.) are given in order to try to improve
239		(the) outlook. keh (.) I'd like to do that after
240		I take a look at you n examine ya.
241	PT 2	mm

Here, at the end of this phase of the visit, the doctor indicates two things: (1) his plan to examine the patient, and (2) his intention to discuss the meaning of having two lymph nodes positive: what the outlook is for that and how the outlook can be improved (lines 233–240). In this way, he clearly displays his knowledge about the import of the patient's condition and forecasts the graveness of her situation by intimating that the outlook could use some improvement. In addition to mentioning his access to her medical records (see excerpt 14), this is another overt display of access to information from the doctor. By projecting this discussion, he casts himself in the role of gatekeeper to the needed information.

Overall, the talk just examined (excerpted from a total of 7 minutes of conversation) provided the details of how these participants orient to one another and cast themselves in the roles of "doctor" and "patient." The doctor treats the patient as someone who either is knowledgeable about her own medical history and current state of health (excerpts 13, 14, 16) or has access to knowledge from an outside source (excerpt 17). By asking her to account for her delay of biopsy, initiating the interrogative sequence, mentioning access to medical records, proposing the physical exam, and projecting an explanation of the patient's diagnosis/prognosis, the doctor both enacts and talks about activities that situate him as someone with institutional rights, responsibilities, and expert knowledge.

For her part, the patient treats the doctor as someone with expertise or knowledge (excerpts 15 and 17) and presents herself as ignorant in the realm of what they both construct as expert medical knowledge (excerpt 17). She asks him to predict her future mental and physical state, focuses on her mispronunciation of a technical term, and does not resist the physical examination.

The purpose of following this interaction in some detail is to show how discourse identities are not fixed or immutable but are oriented to in different ways at different moments in the interaction. I have tried to show thus far how the identities of expert and novice, or service provider and service seeker, are made manifest within the details of the talk and activity. Both parties have moments in which they are experts ratifying the accounts of the other or showing some alignment in their understanding of the facts of the case; "expertise" is not the unique domain of the doctor at all points in the encounter. To be sure, moments of patient expertise are rare in the medical visit, but taking note of such instances enriches our understanding of the doctor-patient relationship. Expertise must be made manifest—displayed or called on—to become a relevant feature of a participant's role in an interaction.

Through a variety of mechanisms, such as information gathering, displayed access to information, third-party reference, self-presentation, and orientation to the "other" as expert, it is evident that participants do continuous work to create and recreate roles within the encounter. The next section examines a particular activity—patient appeals for information—to illustrate how participants manage the sometimes conflicting roles of patient as advice-seeker and doctor as gatekeeper.

4.2 Patient Requests for Information or Guidance

The remainder of this chapter examines excerpts from the rest of the data to support the idea of mutually constructed discourse identities within the office visit. I further suggest that expertise is not simply internal to a person (i.e., the storage of knowledge) but is made manifest or called on or offered up in the to and fro of interaction. People treat one another and themselves as knowledgeable (or not) in various ways. Perhaps the most obvious way is to simply ask someone for assistance by asking for an opinion or information. This conversational action proposes that the co-participant has some expertise or knowledge to provide. This section focuses on patients' requests (through questioning) for information and how those appeals are treated. Thus there are really two issues to tease apart: (1) who gets to ask questions and when, and (2) who is being constituted through the questions as having knowledge.

It has been shown that in general internal medicine consultations, patient questions are dispreferred in that they often fail to elicit answers from the doctor (Frankel, 1989; West, 1983; West & Frankel, 1991). On the surface, that is what appears to be happening in excerpt 15; the patient poses a question only to have the doctor reply with a question. The "turn taking" is recalibrated, perhaps in the service of further information gathering to answer her question, though, as shown, an answer was never forthcoming. I propose that it may not be the patient's question itself that is dispreferred but instead that the sequential placement of a question during phase 3 is dispreferred. This view supports the observation that in general practice consultations (in the Netherlands), "the dispreference for patient-initiated questions seems to be phase specific" (ten Have, 1991, p. 149).

As noted in chapter 3, the oncologists in these data often *invite* the patient to divulge concerns and frame questions at the outset of the clinic visit. This process is often accomplished unproblematically within the first few minutes of the encounter. However, it is notable that some patient concerns articulated in the opening minutes of the encounter, concerns that invite some prediction about prognosis or treatment, are often treated as delayable objects. They are attended to in a way that acknowledges the asking but does not actually answer them. Delaying the patient question is a way in which the doctor displays expertise within, and control over, the encounter. This analysis overlaps with the discussion of the agenda-based nature of these encounters in chapter 3. It is not that there is a dispreference for patient questions per se but, rather, that deferring some types of patient questions may be a way by which doctors establish themselves as controlling the consultation agenda. The doctor thus instantiates him or herself as the expert in terms of what is appropriate information seeking and at which specific times. Because patients rarely contest the doctor's deferral of their questions (rarely pursuing a response) this can be seen as the patient participating in the doctor's control of how and when information is transferred.

There are many examples of patients or their co-present friends and relatives asking questions of the doctor. Depending on where in the sequence of the visit the questions arise and what the topic is, doctors are more or less amenable to answering them. If they arise prior to the physical examination, the doctor seems likely to sidestep the question by postponing, either through initiating a new sequence of questions (as in excerpt 15) or with a promise to get to the matter next, or after the physical exam, or at some unspecified future time (as in excerpts 3 and 4 in chapter 3). This chapter looks more closely at questions that arise prior to the recommendation in phase 5. Questions arising within the recommendation phase are treated rather differently and are analyzed in detail in chapter 5.

In the first example (excerpt 19), Doctor 7's response to Patient 91's query is to delay his reply. He projects an answer to come rather than actually answering her question. The patient has been taking tamoxifen and now wonders if that is appropriate; she has been getting different opinions on what the optimum course of treatment would be. Just prior to the excerpt transcribed, the doctor had mentioned that the major question "right now" is whether or not to give chemotherapy.

Excerpt 19

DR 7 So if it were gonna be done, it should be done (.)
you know (.) reasonably soon.
PT 91 What what is the advantage? Ya know I I think I need
somebody to explain that <u>to</u> me. How much better off
am I going to be if I have chemothera[py.
DR 7 [Yeh.
PT 91 and the tamoxifen.
DR 7 Right. Okay well <u>that</u> that's the next thing I was
gonna get get to.

Here the patient asks a focused question of the doctor (line 60), then continues with a mitigated appeal for an explanation (lines 60–61), then reforms her original question with another direct question (lines 61–62).

The intermediate request (lines 60–61) for assistance/explanation is vitiated in its form. Sandwiched between the two direct questions, it is hedged by the place holder "ya know" followed by repetition of the pronoun "I," the qualifying verb "think" and the generic noun "somebody." This formulation mitigates what could otherwise have been a direct appeal to the co-present doctor (if she had chosen to use a personal pronoun "you" and a stand-alone verb "need" as in "I need for you to explain that to me").

This statement of need, though hedged and qualified, potentially places the doctor in the position as fulfiller of the need. Her appeal to "somebody" is rather vague, but she follows that up with a reformulation ("how much better off will I be") of her initial question. This is an explicit request for information formulated as something to which only the doctor has access.

Why does the patient not simply stop after her initial question "What is the advantage . . .?" (line 60). Based on the talk that preceded, it is known to these participants that the patient has been gathering information and recommendations about adjuvant therapy from a number of doctors. Her follow-up, or statement of need at lines 60–61, refines what she means by her question and may point to the fact that, as yet, no one has actually explained to her satisfaction the advantages of chemotherapy.

The doctor's response, that he was "gonna get get to" that (line 66) proposes that the patient is getting ahead of him. By making the statement, the doctor displays that he has the patient's question in mind. In this way, he moves to present himself as someone who knows what her concerns might be even before she has voiced them. His utterance reasserts his role not only as the one managing the activities but also as the expert prepared with the information and explanations that the patient needs.

In another example of this type (excerpt 20), the doctor has asked the patient about the results of her progesterone receptor test. The patient responds that her progesterone receptors were positive, but she does not recall the exact numerical value.[2] Her husband then asks the significance of the receptors.

Excerpt 20 (HU = Husband)

216	PT 30	But it it was positive.
217	DR 4	Okay. Now=
218	HU 30	=Can can [you uh (.)
219	DR 4	[How are you ah
220	HU 30	expound- that's one of the questions, expound upon
221		the significance of that.

222	DR 4	Yeah [I'll uh
223	PT 30	[He'll get-
224	DR 4	I'll go into that [in a
225	PT 30	[yeah.
226		(2.0)
227	DR 4	in a fair amount of detail.
228	PT 30	[( )
229	DR 4	[Uhhh, what that means. Now, uhm
230		(4.5)
231		You're forty-one?

Again, the doctor is asked directly to address a concern (in this case raised by the patient's husband.) The doctor promises to address the question (line 224) but for the moment turns the agenda to collecting medical history (line 231). Note how the patient, who described herself earlier as a nurse, aligns with the doctor: Her utterance at line 223 looks as though it is on its way to predicting the doctor's statement at line 224. The patient thus cooperates with the doctor in voicing (to her husband) the "promise" that an answer will be forthcoming at the appropriate time. In this way the patient shares with the doctor the institutional role that is usually exclusively the doctor's. She presents herself as a participant in the institution, and it is actually the husband, not the patient, who is being asked to wait.

These excerpts show that the doctor may respond to a patient question with a deferral that promises future response. Patients rarely pursue their questions further after these moves by the doctor, thereby relinquishing their request for information and "accepting" that answers will be forthcoming. But this is not to say that all patient questions that directly request information are deferred. In fact, in four encounters in which questions relating to cancer causation are raised by patients or family members, those concerns are addressed as they arise. This generalization bears verification in similar settings, but for the current data it is clear that concerns about causation are dealt with immediately by the doctors.[3]

In excerpt 21, the patient raises a concern about what may have caused her breast cancer. She explains that she does not smoke or drink and then asks whether it could be the fact of coloring her hair. The patient does pursue further explanation from the doctor by continuing to reformulate her concerns. She accepts the question as finally answered when the doctor tells her that she can continue coloring her hair. And then the doctor returns to the medical history taking they had been involved in just prior.

Excerpt 21

PT 44 Did you- do you thi:nk that putting color on your
hair might have something to do with the cancer?
DR 5 Nope?
PT 44 Because see I don't smoke, I don't drhink, heh .hh
I don't know what does [it.
DR 5 [Well we don't-
PT 44 [( )]
DR 5 [We don't know what] causes breast cancer. We
(.) we don't think smokin or drinkin or hair
coloring has anything to do with it.
PT 44 Oh ya don't?=
DR 5 = [No.
PT 44 [uh huh
DR 5 But we don't know what causes breast [cancer.
PT 44 [Well I
wondered, cause I had read, (.) ya know they said
(1.0) uh:: colorin your hair is bad for ya,=You read
so many things you get so confused. You don't know
what to do.
DR 5 No:: you can keep colorin your hair.
PT 44 Oh, okay, fine.
DR 5 Okay? All right. Uh:: any other pain besides that . . .

The doctor's handling of the patient's question is rather different from how "premature" questions about treatment are handled early in the visit. In excerpt 21 the doctor responds to each of the patient's queries with some kind of answer: "No" responses at lines 140 and 149; in lines 145–147, an explanation that although no one knows what causes breast cancer, the agents named by the patient are not linked to the disease. The doctor provides straightforward answers here; there is no delaying of the patient's concerns to some future point in the consultation. These types of questions regarding causation are always dealt with as they arise, whereas those questions that touch on the efficacy of treatment are deferrable if they arise prior to phase 5 topics (recommendation/ information).

In sum, patient requests for information relate to the question of how discourse identities are established through talk and how the management of participant roles is achieved on a moment-to-moment basis. When patients request information, they are placing the doctor in a position of having some relevant knowledge. Depending on the sequential placement of the patient's question or its topical content, it may be a delayable object.

Patient questions addressed as they arise are those that deal with disease causation. Because these concerns do not pertain to the recommendation to come, they may be attended to as they arise. This highlights the fact that the doctors are orienting to a separate phase of the visit in which treatment-related concerns are to be discussed.

4.3 Patient Preparedness

The previous sections detailed how topic proffering (requests for information) and topic control (delay of answer) are observable behaviors which constitute relevant discourse identities in the adjuvant therapy visits. Patients ask questions to elicit information from doctors, and doctors can delay responses, controlling the sequential placement of topics and activities. The final section of this chapter turns to an important facet of patient identity in these encounters: examining how the patient presents herself as knowledgeable and how doctors participate in that characterization. The identity of "patient" in this setting is not simply one of a person in need of information or service. In these oncologic visits, patients present themselves as seekers of information from other reputable sources. They display an orientation to being well informed and to being open to new information. Doctors ratify patient displays of self-education and cooperate in the construction of the patient as a person prepared and ready to discuss the serious matters at hand, encouraging any signs of patient preparedness.

Looking at the first excerpt in this context (excerpt 22), it is evident that the doctor links the patient's good understanding of the critical treatment issues to the possibility that she (or someone close to her) has been doing "a lot of reading." Reading is an activity that tends to mark people as concerned, inquisitive, and probably factually prepared.

In excerpt 22, the doctor refers to the questions the patient has been asking and remarks on her level of preparation for the visit. His talk in line 64 is responsive to the patient's prior display of access to information. By acknowledging the patient's display of knowledge, the doctor participates in the construction of her as a reasonable and responsible person. He also, therefore, presents himself as a person who can make such a judgment.

Excerpt 22

DR 4 The only thing I can say is that yer yer
questions uh:: indicate a uh (.) a a very good

66 understanding of thee (.) critical issues in this
67 uh: *treatment.*=Have you done a lot of reading? or
68 has your daughter been?
69 PT 83 [Well now there's a big there's a big]
70 DR 4 [I'm just wondering how you] learned so
71 much cause these are very good questions.
72 PT 83 Uh::m they had a big article in the Washington Post
73 about a month ago: on breast cancer, it was very
74 good. I mean it was a three or four page article.
75 Covered most of these subjects.
76 DR 4 Well that's good.
77 PT 83 eh heh heh (it came right along.)
78 DR 4 I'm gonna [hafta I'm gonna hafta
79 PT 83 [(Right around surgery)
80 DR 4 change my biases about the press now. heh yahha
81 know. Because that that that obviously has prepared
82 you to look at the really critical issues in this
83 [decision.
84 PT 83 [*Yeah. Yeah*

In lines 64–68, the doctor notes the patient's apparent preparedness for understanding the issues she will face in deciding about her treatment. He associates her preparedness and understanding with having done "a lot of reading" which he formulates as a question (line 67). He also proposes that the patient's daughter (a nurse, as mentioned earlier in the talk) may have been studying and presumably informing the patient. In either case, his question presupposes that the patient has come to the meeting prepared through having done reading (as opposed, for instance, to talking to people). In lines 81–82, the doctor mentions that the patient is well prepared to look at "the critical issues" involved in making this difficult decision about whether or not to undergo further treatment.

Though I doubt that praise of patient preparedness is unique to the adjuvant therapy discussion, such an activity has not been noted in investigations of other types of medical encounters. In fact, to my knowledge, praise has not been looked at as an interactional resource in any type of talk. Provisionally, then, displaying praise for the patient's preparation to tackle the medical decision may be a resource to show alignment with the patient while still maintaining the doctor's identity as an expert, one who is able to judge another participant's level of understanding.

The next examples demonstrate intersecting aspects of identity made manifest during one encounter. The doctor constructs the patient as a highly informed person and apparently welcomes the difficult challenge of a sophisticated patient. But the patient demurs in the face of this characterization of herself as a near expert and appeals to the doctor to help her sort out her confusion.

This patient is writing a thesis on clinical trials in the treatment of cancer. She mentions this fact early in the talk and the doctor strongly ratifies the patient's display of knowledge as shown in excerpt 23 (line 326). (Some portions of this excerpt are deleted in the interest of preserving patient confidentiality.)

Excerpt 23

296 DR 7 What what are you working on in terms of the- your doctoral
297 program.
298 PT 50 As a matter of fact, I'll be calling you as phhhart of my
299 ☺sthhudy heh huh [heh huh heh huh]
300 DR 7 [I see. That's okay.]
301 PT 50 heh .hhhh ☺You'll have to remember I'm not your patient at
302 all then. Eh heh heh .hhh hhh but we're looking at
303 ((description of study))

.

.

.

307 DR 7 M-hm?
308 PT 50 and (taydarpine),
309 DR 7 Oh yes. Uh huh. ((proper name))
310 PT 50 The co[ncept (also)]
311 DR 7 [( )] Oxford at uh the beginning o::f,
312 PT 50 for ((proper name))'s meeting
313 DR 7 for ((repeats name))'s [meeting.
314 PT 50 [this summer.
315 DR 7 Yes. Yeah.
316 PT 50 Mhm.
317 DR 7 Yeah.
318 PT 50 I just came from Oxford *before (this).* UHHM anyway::,
319 yah uh uh- an I've tried I got the latest- I got the latest on his
320 overviews. for how to (.) treat this. hhh ya know huh huh
321 .hhh ☺just Friday someone called [( )
322 DR 7 [☺All right,
323 PT 50 [.hhh huh huh huh .hhh

324 [(that's fair)
325 ☺so I don't-
326 DR 7 ☺You may be thee most informed patient thaz uh that uh that
327 [we've seen here.
328 PT 50 [hhh heh heh [heh
329 DR 7 [☺And we've seen some pretty informed
330 patients so uhh
331 PT 50 Well there's something coming out for (Schmekelgirdl) next
332 week.=They just had a consensus conference *that's ( ).*
333 ANYWAY uhm (.) that's what I'm working on. Uhhh the
334 ((topic of thesis described))
335 DR 7 Very interesting. I'll be interested in- (.) be glad to help and
336 be interested in uh [seeing your work here.
337 PT 50 [You may be sorry you said that. It's
338 about ten different studies of yours . . .
.
.
.
343 DR 7 ☺There's gonna be plenty of advance notice. Uhh that's uhh
344 that's all paying for. That's uh uhm. ☺Okay. Let's me do this,
345 what I wanna do is just examine you briefly . . .

This interchange establishes that the patient has a high level of understanding about the issues surrounding chemotherapy as an adjuvant treatment for breast cancer. In fact, the doctor characterizes this patient as "the most informed" he has seen (line 326). Throughout the excerpt the doctor and patient move through subtle nuances of collegiality while still maintaining the doctor as the expert. Following is a brief look at some of the details that constitute this interchange as an interplay between a reticent near equal and an expert.

The interchange of the patient's laughter and the doctor's response to it (at lines 299–300) indicates that in their currently relevant roles, recruiting the doctor for the patient's investigation is potentially problematic. The patient initiates laughter (lines 298–299) in the at-the-moment awkward situation of proposing that the doctor be a part of her study. The laughter may indicate that she is managing in the face of this difficulty (Jefferson, 1984b). The doctor's response (line 300) indicates that he has no objection to her proposal, and, in fact, by not taking up her laughter, he presents himself as a recipient who is receptive to the trouble she may be expressing through her laughter (Jefferson, 1984b). In other words, he takes seriously the patient's difficulty in inviting him, the oncologist, to be a subject of her study. His response to her ("That's okay") is hearable as indicating that there is no problem where she might have anticipated one.

Later in the talk, the patient and the doctor display alignment with each other. The doctor's trail-off at line 311 is completed by the patient, and her completion ("for ((proper name))'s meeting") is ratified by the doctor. He further ratifies her information at line 315 ("Yes. Yeah."). Also, these participants exhibit alignment, and even perhaps pursuit of intimacy (Jefferson, Sacks, & Schegloff 1987), by the laughing/smiling together in lines 321–330.

Ultimately, the doctor moves off the topic of the patient's research and preparedness for the current visit by announcing his intention to move the agenda to the physical exam (data not shown). Without knowing the full content of the patient's talk at line 321 it is a bit hard to analyze the doctor's responses at lines 322 and 324, though they look as though they are ratifying what the patient has reported in line 321. Indeed, it is at line 326 that he reports that this patient is probably the most informed he has seen. Being able to make that judgement puts him squarely in the position of evaluating her expertise.

In the next excerpt, later in the conversation, the doctor acknowledges the difficulty that the patient's sophistication can present. It is not clear if he is intimating that her level of understanding makes his job more difficult or if he is acknowledging the difficulties that owning this knowledge could present to her. His expression "just fire away the questions" seems to indicate his acceptance of the challenge of this well-informed patient.

Excerpt 24

367	DR 7	You're sophisticated in terms of your data. It makes
368		it harder, but just fire away the questions.
369	PT 50	I guess that (.) I have stopped reading. There's too
370		much information. And I don't know enough. And I
371		would just like to hear what you have to say about
372		chemotherapy. Your thoughts if there is no node
373		involved.

In line 367 the doctor's characterization of the patient's sophistication is hearably downgraded or refuted by the patient. She characterizes herself as suffering from information overload. She says that she has stopped reading and, at lines 370–373, appeals to the doctor for his opinion on her particular case. This is a fairly subtle negotiation: The patient displays extensive knowledge, not only through her previous questions but also by mentioning the thesis she is working on—prima facie evidence that she is well informed about issues in chemotherapy. Yet she characterizes herself as having overloaded on information and therefore as being at a standstill in her understanding—at a point at which the doctor's help is now needed. So even a person who is an expert in her own right demurs at the doctor's characterization of her as "sophisticated."

The following example further demonstrates that patients choose to present themselves as educable people, though not as *too* informed so as not to usurp the doctor's place. This next patient also makes reference to "reading," which is often treated as a sign of preparedness and ability to confront the issues relevant to adjuvant therapy. In excerpt 25, the patient reports having read about "hard and soft" types of cancer.

Excerpt 25

340	PT 46	I understand there's a hard (.) and a soft. Is
341		there- does that make sense?=I read it in somewhere.
342		I read it in some cancer literature.
343	DR 8	Okay.
344	PT 46	Er the har- the soft and the hard.
345	DR 8	Well, Okay. (.) some breast cancers have calcium in
346		them that makes them hard if you're talking about
347		how they feel.
348	PT 46	No.
349	DR 8	No. You're talking about how fast they grow.
350	PT 46	That's it.
351	DR 8	Okay. They tend . . .

In line 341, the patient appeals to the doctor to confirm her characterization of hard and soft cancer types ("does that make sense?"). She latches onto the request for confirmation of the fact that the source of her understanding comes from something she read (line 341). By latching her talk in this way, she potentially blocks the doctor's response at the transition relevance place to provide an account for her statement. This is not just an idea she came up with, but it is something she surmised from an outside source, something she *read* (her emphasis).

Notably, the patient upgrades the source of her knowledge from having acquired it "somewhere" to having gained it through reading "cancer literature" (line 342). This upgrade casts her understanding in light of a reputable source. Though the talk begins with her presenting herself as a reader of cancer literature, the excerpt ends with the doctor formulating the patient's concerns for her. In the absence of the patient's assent to the doctor's formulation (she simply stops at line 348 with a "No."), the doctor steps in to propose what might be the patient's actual concern about how fast her tumor is growing. In this way, the patient moves to get the doctor to "speak for her." Thus, she sets out to display her capacity for searching out new information through reading but ultimately works to get the doctor to provide the information she is seeking.

Though patients may come to the visit with information from outside sources, they do not present themselves as being in possession of the answers to their questions. They still ask for the doctor's opinion, advice, and information. The patients want information, but they want it in the context of what they already know. This is part of the work that goes on *before* any "new" information on cancer treatment can be transmitted.

4.4 Conclusion

This chapter began with an assertion that to provide a hospitable environment for services to be rendered, individuals must show themselves as capable or expert in the area of concern. The service seeker, for her part, must display a need for the expertise of the co-participant. In essence, the participants may treat one another as either expert or novice through various conversational actions. Doctors present themselves as experts by displaying access to information and how they attempt to control the flow of that information. They cast themselves as gatekeepers to information through the delay of certain types of patient questions. Patients appeal to the doctor as someone who is capable of providing information about their medical status, the significance of particular prognostic factors, or the efficacy of treatment.

Finally, this chapter shows how patients present themselves as educable, reasonable, and flexible. Doctors treat patient preparedness as noteworthy, and as such the patient's educability seems integral to her role as advice seeker. For the unproblematic transfer of service or advice to take place, the recipient must show an ability to understand the information and advice to come. Doctor and patient work cooperatively to establish what the patient knows already, to mark a starting point—which also serves the purpose of framing the encounter in terms of information, facts, and items to be explored. Being reasonable and informed are important for the work that will ensue during the recommendation. At that point the patient must be open to the doctor's logic, the arguments based on medical research, and the slippery concept of the probability of cure. To get in that alignment, any indication that the patient is prepared through reading or through discussions with qualified consultants (family members in the medical profession, other medical personnel) is topicalized by the doctor.

A central question guiding this research is: If these clinic appointments are for discussing adjuvant therapy, then what is all this other talk doing? As noted in chapter 3, establishing and keeping to the "agenda" is related to the conversational achievement of asymmetry and the institutional role of gatekeeper. And this chapter provides more evidence that the talk and actions are partly about displaying expert/novice identities, establishing knowledgeability, creating a context for the transfer of new information (discerning what each participant knows and establishing what they presume the other knows)—which may all contribute to motivating the patient to follow the recommendation to come.

5

The Recommendation

This chapter is concerned with phase 5 of the adjuvant therapy visit: the part of the visit when the doctor delivers and justifies recommendation for further treatment. By "recommendation" I am referring not only to the statement that contains the recommendation but also to the talk surrounding it. The recommendation itself is often a fairly straightforward matter, stated in a sentence such as, "Our recommendation is that you get chemotherapy of some kind." This is not the main work that needs doing though. As evidenced by the extensive discussion (up to 1 hour) surrounding those simple statements, it is clear that the main work to be accomplished is to explain and justify the recommendation, to persuade the patient to take a particular course of action.

The previous chapters illustrated how doctors gain entry into the activity of recommending, how they focus their inquiries on lymph node involvement, how the patient and doctor co-construct an asymmetry of expertise and a service orientation for the visit. This chapter demonstrates how this groundwork supports the recommendation itself. What the analysis in this chapter newly introduces is the role the patient has in constructing her understanding of her situation, and what doctors do in response to that emergent understanding. Though there are rarely any firm decisions about treatment made during the encounter, patients leave the office visit with recommendations to think about. Despite the low rate of on-the-spot agreement to treatment, 80% of these patients do eventually take the advice of the oncologist. Thus the visit is persuasive in some way for the majority of the women seeking advice. Part of the persuasiveness is to be found in the doctors' ability to treat patient concerns as valid and reasonable while still repeating the value of chemotherapy in light of the lurking danger evidenced by positive lymph nodes.

Thinking of a recommendation as a kind of work to be done makes it clear that part of the patient's work is to become an informed person and to make a decision about adjuvant therapy based on her emergent understanding of the evidence being presented. To do this, she must wade through information and sort out its relevance for her particular situation. As discussed in chapter 4, the doctor often notes and praises patients' preparedness and ability to educate themselves. It is during this last phase of their conversation, the point when various aspects of this life-changing decision must be discussed, that the patient's ability to grasp this new knowledge becomes most important. One aspect of the doctor's work is to promote a treatment which, despite its powerful negative effects on the patient's physiology, is not a guaranteed cure. Thus, a conversational dynamic is set up between the patient's job of staying focused on her personal view of the risks and benefits of treatment and the doctor's job of promoting treatment based on risks and benefits for the general population. Management of this dynamic is a central concern of this chapter. Patients in these data do not simply "accept" the doctor's expertise but are active participants in constructing their understanding of the medical situation. As the patient's understanding of the situation emerges through the talk, the doctor works to maintain a balance between not making any guarantees to the patient and still promoting what is considered to be in the patient's best interest. Doctors manage this by tempering patients' overly optimistic conclusions and by fortifying the evidence in favor of treatment when patients are resistant or in doubt as to treatment efficacy.

Section 5.1 looks at the way in which adjuvant chemotherapy is initially justified. Then, section 5.2 looks at patient response to the justification and recommendation. Finally, section 5.3 looks at how these oncology clinic visits are closed.

5.1 Presenting the Rationale for Adjuvant Therapy

Costello (1990) is the only investigation to date that deals specifically, from a conversation analytic point of view, with physician recommendations and patient receipt of those recommendations. As noted by Costello, whose analysis is based on recommendations made in a general medicine clinic, a recommendation is an accountable action; it requires justification (p. 67). Based on the data for the current study, I concur with his observation. In fact, as the following bit of talk indicates, the doctor is oriented to the recommendation as an action requiring justification.

Excerpt 26 (from PT 76 and DR 4)

235	DR 4	The:: the <u>bottom</u> li:ne of my recommendation would be to
236		add chemotherapy. To the tamoxifen.
237		(2.5)
238		And, having said that, let me go back and *uh try and
239		justify that recommendation for you.*

Here, the doctor characterizes the justification as something that would normally precede a recommendation, as in line 238 he says that he will "go back" and justify it. Indeed, the rationale for adjuvant treatment is most often presented at the outset of phase 5, before any recommendation has been made. This presentation occurs in just over half of the encounters, as discussed in this section. In other words, prior to even telling a patient what the next course of action should be, the doctor may first cover information that supports the upcoming recommendation for adjuvant therapy. The oncologist often relates the history of how breast cancer has been treated in the past, the mechanics of metastasis, and the risks of recurrence based on lymph node involvement. These prerecommendation justifications take the shape of a cooperatively maintained extended doctor turn which, in these data, lasts anywhere from 2 minutes to 15 minutes.

Receipt by the patient of the prerecommendation justification takes many forms: Patients simply accept the rationale as presented (and the associated recommendation), they draw conclusions about their chances for a disease-free future, they ask questions to clarify specific bits of information embedded within the justification, or they may refute statements made by the doctor and thereby resist both the justification and the subsequent recommendation. All these patient responses are exemplified in section 5.2 of this chapter.

In the current section, we look only at how oncologists first attempt to justify the use of adjuvant therapy. The recommendation statement can precede or follow this justification or even be embedded within it.

The excerpts in this section are examples of justifications whose rhetorical structure and informational content are quite common in the data. The oncologists often lead up to the recommendation to use chemotherapy by using some slight variations on the following sequence: (1) establishing that surgery was considered acceptable treatment in the past; (2) proposing the notion that residual, undetectable cancer cells can still reside in the body; (3) asserting that positive lymph nodes are markers of residual disease; and (4) reporting that chemotherapy has been shown to be effective for treating residual disease.

The apparent trajectory of these arguments is to conclude that chemotherapy will be of value in the patient's particular case. To illustrate this, we begin with a detailed discussion of Doctor 2's extended turn with Patient 2 at the outset of phase 5. This discussion constitutes a pre-recommendation justification.

In excerpts 27–29, the doctor is laying out the rationale for treatments beyond surgery. Surgery, which is the excision of the tumor and proximal tissue and lymph nodes, constitutes primary treatment of the cancer. Adjuvant therapies (chemotherapy, hormone therapy, radiation) are named as such because they are additional or secondary treatments. Here, the oncologist projects an explanation of breast cancer in general, which leads, essentially, to information on the importance of lymph node involvement as a prognostic tool for assessing the risk of disease recurrence.

Excerpt 27

624 DR 2 Well? let me explain a couple things to you. about (.)
625 breast cancer in general an an your case in particular.
626 In general,
627 (2.2)
628 breast cancer is a disease that we know (.) tends to
629 spread early. an:d (.) it's a disease that in the old
630 days the feeling was that if you uh (.) if you got it
631 out and you got the lymph nodes out the:n that was
632 basically *the best you can do.*

((DR relates the discovery that patients with lymph node involvement tended to have their cancer recur.))

642 DR 2 an:d (.) it was clearly these people who had
643 negative lymph nodes. none a the lymph nodes involved,
644 had about an eighty percent chance of never having

645 their breast cancer come back in their lives. (....)
646 And it depends somewhat on how many <u>nodes</u> are involved.

At lines 624–625, the doctor projects an explanation of breast cancer "in general" and the patient's case "in particular." He starts with the general by saying that breast cancer is a disease that tends to spread early. Notice that the doctor has not formulated this as a simple statement of fact; rather, he has placed himself within a plurality of *knowers of this fact*. The formulation "we know" (line 628) marks this talk about "breast cancer in general" as neither a personal opinion of his nor his personal knowledge—it is something known by more than one person, adding weight to the assertion. As noted by Drew and Heritage (1992), the pronoun "I" is somewhat less institutionally weighted than the "we" form. So, by choosing the pronoun form "we," the doctor achieves a closer alignment with the institution, placing himself within the aggregate knowledge base of the medical profession. In this way, he presents himself as an expert member of the institution.

This "knowing" about breast cancer becomes contrasted with what Doctor 2 says in lines 629–630, "in the old days the feeling was that . . ." This impersonal construction removes the content of the utterance from the realm of the doctor's personal experience. This is not couched as "I felt" or "we felt" but simply as an impersonal report of prior practice. Note that any reference to knowledge is absent, he just reports the "feeling" of that time. In essence, the doctor presents the option of "surgery only" as one associated with a bygone era, implicitly contrasted with current thinking which is knowledge-based, the era with which he had just associated himself. To this point, the patient has only undergone surgery for breast cancer; this visit with the oncologist is to discuss further treatment options. Therefore, at this point in the talk, the patient is presented with the fact that her treatment thus far is a treatment of the "old days."

Following these assertions—that breast cancer is a disease that spreads early, and that it was originally treated surgically only—the doctor's talk develops into a history of the discovery that evidence of tumor in the lymph nodes means that "microscopic bits" of cancer have spread into the body and can cause recurrence (data parenthetically characterized in the excerpt). He then begins developing a topic in which he explains that the chance of recurrence is related to the number of positive lymph nodes (lines 644–646).

In the talk so far, the patient's only vocal contribution has been one continuer. She has ceded the floor to the doctor at each opportunity, participating in his projected explanation. In the continuation of this talk, at line 648 in excerpt 28, however, she speaks up for the first time (about 90 seconds into phase 5) to reiterate that she had two positive nodes. This fact is known to the doctor. Not only is the information in her medical record, but he elicited this information from the patient earlier when asking her about her understanding of her condition (see chapter 4, excerpt 18). The doctor has been adhering to his projected activity of talking about "breast cancer in general" and now the patient attempts to move him to her "case in particular"—the other projected aspect of his talk.

Excerpt 28

646		And it depends somewhat on how many nodes are involved.
647		[If you had-
648	PT 2	[Well I had two.=
649	DR 2	=If you have one to three nodes, (.) you have a::
650		pretty significant chance of it coming back. probably
651		in the range of ah
652		(1.2)
653		forty fifty percent (.) roughly.
654		(0.6)
655		Now:
656		(1.0)
657		if ya have more than (.) four nodes positive then you
658		have a real high chance of it comin back.
659		(1.0)
660	PT 2	mm=

At the end of line 646, there is a convergence of syntactic and prosodic completion, a transition relevance place (TRP) where a next speaker could take a turn without disrupting the talk (Ford & Thompson, 1996; Sacks et al., 1974). Though there have been many such TRPs in this extended explanation, interestingly it is at this point that the patient chooses to take a turn. There is nothing unusual about her cooperation thus far in the doctor's extended turn; it is actually expectable recipient behavior given his earlier projection of an explanation. But she uses the resource of the TRP at the end of line 646 to reiterate that she had two nodes involved. In a sense she interrupts his explanation of the general facts about lymph node involvement, to bring the discussion around to her particular case. But her attempt fails. The overlap (lines 647–648) suggests that the doctor is still orienting to his turn as being in progress. His turn (at line 649) is clearly a display of "turn continuing" in that it repeats both syntactically and prosodically the beginning of the sentence that was overlapped, in this case the *if*-clause conditional (Local, 1992; Schegloff, 1987). The doctor is pursuing the line of talk in which he is presenting the known probabilities of recurrence. By restarting his turn with the *if* clause, the doctor displays that he is still in the middle of his projected explanation.

After the patient comes in with her contribution at the TRP, the doctor reformulates the verb form ("had" becomes "have"), though he chooses not to focus on the patient's particular case. He continues with his hypothetical *if*-clause construction, repairing only the tense marking, but does not abandon the hypotheticality of what he is saying. The doctor could have said, in orienting to the patient's reiteration of her node status, that "with two nodes you have 40–50% chance of recurrence," yet he chooses not to specify at two nodes. He gives her the range within which she fits: one to three nodes. She must infer that she fits into the 40–50% chance of recurrence group. The patient's inference that her chances for survival are "good" comes later in the talk and is discussed in section 5.2.2. Here, the doctor clearly does not relinquish control of the rhetorical shape of the explanation in progress and pursues his listing of alternative scenarios despite the patient's contribution that she had two positive nodes.

The doctor's stance toward his current activity is arguably one of describing general guidelines for probabilities of recurrence; he is not engaging in the particularities of the patient's case. At this point, he is providing her with resources that might lead to a conclusion about the need for further treatment. He begins filling in that piece of the syllogism as he proceeds with the next bit of talk:

Excerpt 29

679	DR 2	Now, what people have done is treated people with
680		chemotherapy, afterwards,

In line 679, he introduces the notion of using chemotherapy to treat people with some evidence of residual disease. He makes this report using a generic statement (lines 679–680), "now, what people have done is treated people with chemotherapy." This statement is rather broad: The doctor mentions neither "women" (the subgroup of "people" most relevant to the patient's illness) nor "oncologists/doctors" (the subgroup of people who treat with chemotherapy). He is talking here in the most general way about people treating other people with chemotherapy. This talk works to maintain his stance of providing general guidelines within which the patient may fit herself. He is not explicitly doing that work for her. Nonetheless, his recommendation that the patient undergo chemotherapy is incipient here—though not fully expressed, the implication could be drawn by the patient. The next section looks further at this excerpt as the patient's response to the rationale for treatment (based on her two positive lymph nodes) is examined in detail. For now, just the shape of the oncologists' initial justification is being reviewed.

The following two excerpts (30 and 31) are further examples of how a trajectory of arguments similar to what was laid out previously is followed by other oncologists. The first excerpt follows the common line of argumentation as described earlier. The patient participates in this extended turn, which ultimately lasts about 5.5 minutes. Here, excerpt 30 just presents the first minute or so of talk by the doctor.

Excerpt 30 (from PT 43 and DR 7)

327	DR 7	When you l:ook at (.) uhm a breast cancer, uhm
328		what what ya you do is ya say well we've got to
329		remove the tumor, and that's what was done. Uhhm
330		the tumor was removed, uh the remaining (.) uh
331		tissues in the area were removed, as well as the
332		uh lymph nodes. A::nd as I said ten years ago you
333		would have been to:ld uhhh that's it. Ya know (.)
334		don't worry about it. *( )*. The problem
335		with that is, that (.) in a f:air number of cases
336		of uh women with breast cancer, uhhm the disease
337		can recur, a::nd what we think is going on, is
338		there could be:: little nests of cells that can't
339		be seen with +any test ya do, bone scans, or
340		whatever+ there could be in different areas of the
341		body, but the body itself may take care of with
342		its own immune mechanisms. But that in certain
343		patients it (.) they they will develop into:
344		actual metastases. Now. How do you select out (.)
345		of all the patients with breast cancer: who's most
346		likely to have this problem.=And ya do that, with-
347		the single best way is looking at the lymph nodes.
348		The size of the tumor is a factor, uhhhm but the
349		lymph nodes uhhm if the lymph nodes were all
350		negative, the size may be a more important

factor.=What I was tryin to tell ya before in view
of the fact that your lymph nodes were positive
that really becomes almost a dominant factor.
Uhhm and given that, we know that in women who
have (.) uhm lymph nodes involved that there's a
greater chance (.) for (.) recurrence in the
future.=Therefore (.) something should be done
now. And in women in your (.) age group, the
results have been very encouraging with the use of
chemotherapy.

Here, Doctor 7 begins by recapturing for Patient 43 the fact that the tumor itself, surrounding tissue, and lymph nodes have been removed (lines 330–332). He relates this to what was considered standard treatment in the past—"ten years ago" (line 332).

The doctor identifies a problem with that older style of treatment in that the disease recurs in some women (lines 334–337). Then, at line 337, he introduces a theory ("what we think is going on . . .") that residual cells reside in the body but are undetectable (lines 338–340). He then poses a "rhetorical question" in lines 344–346; that is, a question that the addressee is not necessarily expected to answer. His question simply moves the argument along as the answer is clearly not in the patient's domain of knowledge (the "you" is arguably not meant to refer to her). And, structurally, the question is posed without a pause following it where a pause might indicate a space for response. The patient does not initiate an answer and, in fact, the doctor "rushes through" (Schegloff, 1987) the possible transition space at the end of his question to continue his extended turn.

This rhetorical question, bounded by the rush through, sets up a framework in which the doctor is providing an answer to his own question. In this way, Doctor 7 delivers the information that lymph node involvement is the surest indicator of the extent of residual disease. He mentions finally at lines 358–360 that chemotherapy has had encouraging results for women in this patient's age group. From here, the doctor moves on to discuss particular options within the range of chemotherapeutic drugs. The doctor's turn continues for another 4.5 minutes until the patient raises a question about whether or not chemotherapy is followed up by radiation therapy. In total, then, his extended turn lasts about 10 minutes. A distinctly different turn length from those in all previous phases of these encounters.

In the talk we have looked at thus far, from both Doctor 2 and Doctor 7, the oncologists are presenting themselves as having access to historical information about the treatment of breast cancer and about effectiveness of chemotherapy for reducing the risk of disease recurrence. Patients cooperate in these extended turns by holding their questions, and they cooperate in the construction of the doctor's expertise by not refuting any of the information being offered. Patients rarely contradict or corroborate any of the facts being presented. In excerpt 28, when Patient 2 reiterated that she had two positive nodes, the doctor ignored her contribution in favor of continuing his projected explanation. Her contribution was not treated as relevant at that point in the unfolding justification. Thus, not only is it rare for patients to show "expertise," but when they do, as in this case, the doctor may treat their contributions as inconsequential.

The final example reviewed is from a visit I recorded. This hospital is geographically separated (by over 1,000 miles) from the hospital where the rest of the data were collected. Yet the format of the justifications is strikingly similar. I was in the room at the initiation of the encounter as the doctor and patient reviewed the meaning of her 13 positive lymph nodes. Due to the constraints on audiotaping the encounter, the tape recorder did not get turned on quickly enough so we miss the opening of their discussion. The doctor and patient had talked on the phone prior to this visit and had seen each other once before; this accounts for the deletion of phases 2 and 3 in their encounter. Phase 4, the physical exam, occurs later in the talk. Despite these formal differences from most of the rest of the data, we see in the following excerpt how the doctor's justification follows a similar trajectory in terms of rhetorical structure and information ordering as outlined previously.

Excerpt 31

DR 1	[microphone noise] there's a a possibility that
	there may have some cancer cells have escaped beyond
	[microphone noise]
PT 101	mm
DR 1	And we do know that the probability and the chances
	of it are pretty /high/
	(1.0)
	Now ih in the old days we used to sort of say, w
	let's just watch it and ya know, the surgeon's taken
	everything out the bone scan an everything is okay
PT 101	mm=
DR 1	=but that just means ya know that that we'll jus see

13		what happens. And there still is a chance without
14		any (.) ya know anything else that your your tumor
15		(.) you're doing fine. But if you were to sorta take
16		a hundred patients like yourself(.) ya know the
17		chances of coming back would be pretty /high/ the
18		figures are maybe (.) nine outta ten
19	PT 101	mm
20	DR 1	so (.) it means that it's pretty serious *in terms
21		of that.* Now (.) now that's sort of the the bad
22		news the question is what can we do: with that
23		*now.* The the cancer uh ya know now we have some
24		treatments or medicines that uh ya know we know help
25		in terms of keeping it from coming *back.*
26	PT 101	mm
27	DR 1	*Now* the treatments basically range from
28		chemotherapy which is a (.) a (.) ahhhhh ya know
29		intravenous injections and pills. And then also to
30		drugs like tamoxifen, which is a a drug that does ya
31		know works on the tumor cells and keeps them from
32		growing.
33	PT 101	mm

Here again, the doctor introduces the notion of residual disease (lines 1–3). He contrasts the knowledge of the "old days" (line 8) with what kind of treatment is "now" available (lines 23–25). The doctor moves on to discuss the various treatment options without resistance from the patient.

What these three excerpts illustrate is how the oncologists in these data begin phase 5 activities with a general rationale for the utilization of adjuvant therapy. The argumentation usually follows from some indication of how breast cancer was treated in the past, to the observation that certain patients had their cancer recur, which led to using chemotherapy to help reduce the risk of recurrence. By covering this historical information, doctors not only display access to that specialized knowledge but also imply that there have been advances in the treatment of breast cancer over the years. Thus the patient is presented with the inferable notion that the treatments being currently recommended are the result of long experience and therefore refined and probably worthwhile. Those cases in which the recommendation is stated first and then followed by a justification seem more common when the recommendation is being sought as a second opinion. As Doctor 4 says to Patient 27, who has come for a second opinion, "So that there's no beating around the bush here, uh:: you you should have this treatment" (data not shown). A statement he then goes on to justify.

As noted, these initial doctor turns in phase 5 often go uninterrupted by the patient. This does not mean, however, that patients simply stay quiet during phase 5. On the contrary, the next section looks at how patients come in to this discussion of adjuvant therapy. Their receipt of the recommendation, or their receipt of certain aspects of the justification, make this part of phase 5 a crucial intersection for observing doctor and patient orientation to the work they each have to do in these clinic visits.

5.2 Patient Receipt of the Recommendation and Doctor Response

As mentioned previously, patient response to the justification or recommendation takes various forms. Patients either simply accept the information and recommendation without resistance or draw conclusions aloud about the information being offered, ask for clarifications, or even resist some aspect of the doctor's presentation. Each of these types of patient response is exemplified here along with an analysis of the doctor's handling of that response. In each example it is apparent that the doctor is trying to balance between not guaranteeing a cure and still promoting treatment. The discussion of patient receipt of recommendations begins with a look first at an unproblematic encounter. I call this "passive receipt" because the patient never raises an objection to the justification or the recommendation. The doctor reinforces the patient's positive disposition toward chemotherapy by treating that choice as rational and sensible.

5.2.1 Passive Receipt: Patient 60 and Doctor 6

In this encounter, the patient is positively disposed to treatment, perhaps even before hearing the doctor's arguments, and she questions neither the recommendation nor the justification leading up to or following it. The oncologist makes the recommendation to get chemotherapy after a 16-minute extended turn in which she has talked about the rationale for treatment and the main treatment options. The oncologist recommends chemotherapy to the patient, though she leaves open an option of radiation treatment and no chemotherapy.

Following some information about the timing of radiation, the patient is asked if she has any questions. Patient 60 responds that she wonders whether she can be treated closer to home; this response seems to be an implicit acceptance of the recommendation for chemotherapy. Explicit acceptance appears in lines 591–592 of excerpt 32.

Excerpt 32

585	DR 6	I can think of several people in the (city name)
586		area that I could phone up and see if they'd be
587		willing to take you on.
588	PT 60	Nk.
589	DR 6	And see what they have to say about that. Okay?
590		would that be better for you?=
591	PT 60	=Yeah. I'm ya know personally (.) ya know would
592		like to have the treatment,
593	DR 6	m-hm?=
594	PT 60	=because it runs in my family,
595	DR 6	m-hm?
596	PT 60	And like I said I (meet)=
597	DR 6	= [m-hm?
598	PT 60	[with my mother she went the [first
599	DR 6	[m-hm?
600	PT 60	method.
601	DR 6	[m-hm,
602	PT 60	[and
603	DR 6	((cough))
604	PT 60	ya know in two years
605	DR 6	[yeah.
606	PT 60	[she was gone.

At line 592, the patient expresses her preference for being treated with chemotherapy and then (lines 594–606) provides an account for that preference: Her mother did not take any treatment beyond surgery and died 2 years after diagnosis (lines 598–606). The "first method" that the patient refers to in lines 598–600 is the option of taking no treatment.

As the discussion continues, the doctor takes up the patient's positive attitude toward therapy to reinforce that treatment option. The doctor prefaces this by putting her medical opinion in perspective saying that she would not "get up on a soap box" and tell the patient she had to take chemotherapy. Even though this patient displays herself to be fully accepting of the recommendation, she is still cautioned by the doctor about the nonstandardness of what is being recommended (data not shown). This cautioning allows the doctor to keep a balanced footing regarding treatment. The doctor promotes chemotherapy while counterbalancing that recommendation with a few caveats. In this way, she presents herself as being honest about the options she has been discussing, showing herself to be balanced and "up front" about the negative aspects of her recommendation. Nonetheless, at the end of a long turn, the doctor reaffirms her opinion in favor of treatment and couches it as "a reasonable thing to do." Excerpt 33 is the close of the doctor's turn.

Excerpt 33

630 DR 6 Uhm, but given (.) your attitude and given the
631 situation you find yourself in, I think it would
632 be a reasonable thing to do.

Here, the doctor has linked the patient's attitude (which is expressly positive toward chemotherapy) and her "situation" (the constellation of prognostic factors and her family history) to the use of chemotherapy (indexed by the pronoun "it" in line 631) as a "reasonable thing to do" (line 632). She casts that course of action in light of rationality. By doing this, the doctor treats the patient's preference as sensible. This works to both praise the patient and reassure her that she made a proper decision. This decision is placed squarely on the patient's shoulders, as shown in the next excerpt.

Toward the end of the consultation, the doctor continues with an endorsement of the patient's choice to be treated. (The talk receipted at line 709 in excerpt 34, is relative to a preceding topic of gathering up some records to send with the patient.)

Excerpt 34

709 PT 60 Okay.=
710 DR 6 =And <u>my</u> account. And I'll uhm talk to some of my
711 oncology friends down here and see if I can find
712 somebody whose (.) thinking is (.) compatible with
713 yours.
714 PT 60 m-hm

.

.

.

728 PT 60 Yeah I feel I've really feel comfortable about
729 being [treated

DR 6	[Okay.
PT 60	Cause like I [said
DR 6	[Yeah,
PT 60	by going through it (.)
DR 6	ye [ah
PT 60	[<u>with</u> my mother and-
DR 6	Yeah well you've seen the worst (.)
PT 60	m-hm,
DR 6	scenario. And and I think that it makes sense to
	try and do everything you can at the beginning to
	try and prevent that from happening.

In lines 712–713, the doctor again treats the patient's choice to pursue further treatment as a rational choice, proposing that the patient find an oncologist near the patient's home whose "thinking" is compatible with the patient's. It is now the patient's, not the doctor's, thinking that is being aligned with. In this way, the decision has been shifted into the realm of the patient's choice and the doctor is now in a position to reinforce that shift. At line 738 the doctor refers to the "sense" it makes to do everything one can early in the process to prevent future difficulties. She again takes the opportunity to reinforce the patient's positive attitude toward further therapy.

Oncologists in these data are often times trying to persuade patients to undergo treatments that are highly toxic and not guaranteed to cure. The decision to undergo treatment is, however, ultimately up to the patient's interpretation of the complex facts presented to her. By taking the opportunity to praise the sensibleness of the patient's decision, Doctor 60 is reinforcing both the patient's agency in making the final decision and, in this doctor's view, making a smart decision.

Very rarely, however, do these unfold with so little input from the patient. More commonly, patients raise concerns and questions as the oncologists bring forth information. The next three excerpts reveal moments in which patients draw conclusions about the efficacy of therapy for their particular case. As I proposed at the outset of this chapter, part of the patient's work in this oncology visit is to come to terms with the information and recommendation for her particular case. As patients go about making sense of the information being presented to them, doctors respond to promote what can be characterized as cautious optimism.

As shown in the following examples, one patient's optimistic conclusion about the curative power of chemotherapy is tempered by the oncologist, but so is her pessimistic conclusion. In the second case, the patient's request for clarification elicits a long response from the doctor in which he navigates between not guaranteeing complete cure but still encouraging the use of treatment. The oncologists in these data attempt to maintain this balance throughout the conversation, unless, as shown in the final case, the patient strongly resists their recommendation. In that instance, invoking the roles of "doctor" and "patient" becomes a resource for persuading the patient to consider further treatment.

5.2.2 Tempering Patient Response: Patient 2 and Doctor 2

In the first example, where a doctor tempers a patient's response, Patient 2 draws an optimistic conclusion about the efficacy of chemotherapy and then displays some pessimism. The doctor maneuvers between these patient inferences about the efficacy of treatment.

Previously, in excerpt 28, Patient 2 tried to insert the information about her lymph node status ("Well I had two") into the doctor's general discussion of risks of recurrence based on node involvement. The attempt failed at that point. The doctor was laying out the mechanisms of cancer spread and the risks of recurrence based on lymph node involvement. In excerpt 35 the conversation picks up at the doctor's first mention of the use of chemotherapy as a treatment for people with evidence of residual disease.

Excerpt 35

679 DR 2 now, what people have done is treated people with
680 chemotherapy, afterwards,
.
.
.
698 and hopefully (.) down the line prevents (.) that
699 from *coming back (.) and (.) causing problems
700 [*(later)*
701 PT 2 [well with only two then I have a good chan::ce?
702 right?=
703 DR 2 =you have a good chance, but ya have still have a
704 significant chance +like I said you have probably a+
705 (.) forty fifty percent chance of the tumor
706 still comin back.

In line 679, the doctor introduces the notion of using chemotherapy to treat people with some evidence of residual disease (i.e., people with positive lymph nodes). As mentioned in the discussion of excerpt 29, this type of statement is not uncommon in the data; it is a broad report on how using chemotherapy is an advisable treatment for people with positive lymph nodes. I noted earlier that this required an inference on the part of the patient that chemotherapy would be advisable in her situation.

At line 701 the patient takes what the doctor so far has been saying to infer, in fact, that her chances for survival are good—because she has only two positive nodes. Here, qualifying that it is "only" two nodes, she displays an optimistic understanding that this should mean she has a "good chance" of no further problems. Her interrogative tag "right?," which she tacks on to her assertion, invites agreement from the doctor. There is no gap between her talk and the doctor's response; in fact, his utterance is latched to the patient's, which could mark this as a firm agreement (Pomerantz, 1984, p. 69). However, the doctor continues with a contrasting statement, "but you still have a significant chance . . ." (lines 703–704), formulating the whole utterance as a weak agreement.

It has been well grounded in ordinary conversation that participants tend first to shape their turns toward agreement with co-participants' positive or negative assessments and then to introduce any disagreement (Pomerantz, 1984; Sacks, 1987): a kind of "yes, but . . ." phenomenon. In this case, the doctor is using that resource in balancing the risks and benefits at this important moment. The patient is on the lookout for clues that her situation is not dire—she reasonably draws that conclusion based on what she has been hearing and then looks to the doctor to confirm it. The doctor firmly agrees with the patient that she has a good chance, aligning briefly with that optimism, but then reintroduces the "significant" chance of recurrence. He tempers her optimism, underscoring that she is still at a 40% or 50% risk of the cancer returning. In this way, he displays that the patient has drawn a reasonable conclusion, displays his receipt of her concern, but still cautions her. His job is to persuade the patient of the usefulness of chemotherapy without guaranteeing any positive outcome. To do this, he acknowledges her optimistic conclusion and reintroduces the lurking danger of the 50% recurrence rate.

As the talk continues (excerpt 36), the patient focuses on that potential danger and draws another inference about chemotherapy, now pessimistically voicing concern that it cannot completely clear up all the residual cancer cells that may be present in her system (lines 716–717).

Excerpt 36

PT 2 mm.
DR 2 despite the fact that there are only two. OUR: (.)
hope would be that if we did the chemotherapy we
would decrease that chance even more.
(1.0)
probably:
(0.8)
what we know of old studies that have been done with
this probably by half the [chances-
PT 2 [chemotherapy doesn't
clear it (altogether then).
DR 2 well it (.) it doesn't guarantee the fact that you-
it won't come back.
PT 2 [mm
DR 2 [it decreases the chance that it will come back.
and that's why we'll recommend it. to most people.
(0.6)

At line 718, the doctor again orients toward agreement with the patient, this time with her negative assessment, but here he displays somewhat delayed agreement, prefacing his utterance with "well" and the repetition of "it." His initial agreement allows for the fact that there are no guarantees, but he mitigates the statement by highlighting, with word stress, that chemotherapy "decreases" the chance of recurrence (line 721). Again, the patient does the work of drawing a conclusion based on what she has been hearing—this time an arguably negative assessment of the efficacy of chemotherapy—and the doctor works to temper that negativity and promote his belief that chemotherapy is recommendable.

At line 722, the doctor links the statement that chemotherapy decreases the chance of recurrence with the statement that chemotherapy is generally recommended. After the next TRP (in line 722, after "it".), there is no uptake by the patient of the doctor's remark, and he works to qualify it by formulating his next utterance as a grammatical continuation (Ford, Fox, & Thompson, 1996). By adding the prepositional phrase "to most people" to the statement that chemotherapy is generally recommended, the doctor still has not told the patient that she will also be recommended to take chemotherapy, though a few lines later he does do that. At that point, there is no verbal sign of uptake from the patient and the topic is cooperatively closed (data not shown). It is not unusual to pass from the justification of the recommendation to other topics, particularly treatment side effects, without explicit acceptance of the recommendation.

Up to this point, the doctor has provided the patient with certain resources for decision making: the mechanics of cancer spread through the lymph nodes, probabilities of recurrence based on the number of positive lymph nodes, the fact that chemotherapy is recommended to most people to decrease the chance of recurrence. The patient has been responsibly drawing some personal conclusions from the doctor's presentation and the doctor has softened or tempered each of those. When the patient's inference is too optimistic, the doctor cautions her; when her inference is too pessimistic, he provides some encouragement. The patient works to clarify her understanding relative to her particular case—what her individual chances are for disease-free survival. For his part, the doctor maneuvers between an effort to avoid guarantees and still promoting an increased chance of survival.

In the next case, however, the doctor counterbalances his *own* talk to keep on an even footing between encouraging treatment while not making any guarantees about outcomes. In this next case, the patient seeks clarification of a particular point.

5.2.3 Working toward Balance within an Extended Turn: Patient 53 and Doctor 7

In excerpt 37, Patient 53 draws a tentative conclusion, based on the talk so far, that chemotherapy will be a definitive cure, destroying any cancer cells currently in her system. The doctor negates her conclusion and clarifies that there is no such guarantee from the treatment. His talk continues, however, to encourage the patient toward adjuvant treatment. Interestingly, the doctor points to the very talk that they are having as an indicator of the uncertainties surrounding the use of chemotherapy.

Excerpt 37

351	PT 53	Okay, so the chemotherapy that I- I would get
352		(.)wouldn't (.) really
353		(2.0)
354		*ahhhh dunno if I understood that* .hh wouldn't
355		stop it from (.) from getting it in the other
356		breast, but=

357	DR 7	=Right.=
358	PT 53	=if there was cancer cells right now in my body,
359	DR 7	Right.=
360	PT 53	=it would definitely,
361	DR 7	WELL IT WOULDN'T- again I uh buh I (.) I CAN'T say
362		it would definitely. It's the best thing we know,
363		and it's certainly been (.) helpful in significant
364		numbers of patients.=It's not- (.) I can't- eh no
365		doctor- I mean if if this were a situation where I
366		er- where I could tell you it's a hundred percent
367		chance that this'll work, and no side effects,
368		then I'd- ya know I'd probably: what I'd probably
369		do: is uh have much shorter conversations and
370		just have people line up (.) and get it. The
371		situation i::s uhm I think it has a good chance of
372		helping ya, uhhm there'd probably be some side
373		effects but not (.) ya know: most patients find it
374		very (.) tolerable and they can they can deal with
375		it very effectively. Uhm AND I think in your case
376		at least it's worthy of (.) your consideration.
377	PT 53	mm-

From lines 351 to 360, the patient provides her understanding of what she has heard so far. Her remark at line 354 ("ahhh dunno if I understood that") is lower in amplitude than the surrounding talk and is sandwiched (grammatically) between "wouldn't really" (line 352) and a repeat of "wouldn't" in "wouldn't stop" (lines 354–355). The two "wouldn'ts" have the same amplitude and pitch. This seems to fit a pattern noted by Local (1992), which marks the "I don't know" as parenthetical. The parenthetical remark along with the 2-second pause preceding it delays the content of the patient's utterance and marks ahead of time that her understanding is tentative. The intonation on the patient's term "definitely" is hearable as a trail-off—it leaves the door open for some correction or completion by the doctor. In this way, by the tentativeness of her question and by the trail-off at the end of her utterance, the patient treats the doctor as an expert, as the one able to clarify the situation she has been trying to understand. She apparently invites the doctor to complete her sentence.

At line 361 the doctor negates the emerging proposition that chemotherapy would definitely eradicate any residual cancer cells. His turn continues, however, with the statement that chemotherapy is the "best" answer to the patient's problems in that it has helped many patients (lines 362–364).

But the doctor doesn't end his turn on this positive note about the helpfulness of chemotherapy. At line 364 he rushes through the TRP after "patients" to reintroduce the uncertainties of the therapies he has been describing. Thus he moves to balance the optimistic conclusion just made with the reality that there are no guarantees. The doctor initiates three negative statements at line 364. The third one ("no doctor") is hearable as an upgrade of the second one ("I can't-"). He orients to the patient's reference to something "definitive" in the cure (see lines 360 and 362), but he can't provide that kind of promise. The repeated self-repairs may indicate some resistance to making absolute statements such as "I can't guarantee" or "no doctor can guarantee." He stops just short of making those incipient negative statements and changes the direction of his talk. He proposes a hypothetical situation to illustrate that if there were a 100% certainty of cure, he would not need to talk to patients. Thus the very act of speaking with the patient, as he currently is, signals the uncertain nature of the treatments being recommended.

At lines 370–371 the currently ongoing activity is explicitly contrasted with the hypothetical situation when the doctor begins his utterance with "The situation i::s" and then goes on to reiterate that chemotherapy is worthy of the patient's consideration. Note that choosing chemotherapy is not presented as a foregone conclusion. The patient is named as the one who must make that decision.

The overall progression of this sequence is that the patient's cautiously optimistic conclusion about the curative power of chemotherapy is at first corrected by the doctor, then that correction is gradually tempered. Thus, by the end of the doctor's extended turn, he has navigated between not guaranteeing complete cure while still encouraging the use of treatment.

By counterbalancing what they themselves say (as previously) or what the patients are concluding (as with Patient 2 and Doctor 2), oncologists artfully manage patient concerns in light of the inescapable uncertainties of adjuvant treatment. Doctor 2 first tempered the patient's optimistic conclusion about her chances of survival, then moved to reinforce the value of chemotherapy when Patient 2 expressed concern about efficacy. Doctor 7 took Patient 53's cautiously optimistic understanding about definitive treatment and corrected it, though proceeded to balance and rebalance his presentation until in the end he encouraged the use of chemotherapy.

While patients are trying to make sense of the information they are receiving in terms of their own particular case, the doctors must negotiate around the uncertainties of the treatments they are proposing. These patients were trying to make sense of the information being presented to them, and they were drawing some reasonable conclusions. In the final example in this section, we see what happens when a patient resists the doctor's presentation, calling into question his expertise.

5.2.4 Patient Resistance: Patient 70 and Doctor 4

In this encounter, Patient 70 does not draw any conclusions based on what she has been hearing in the talk so far (as did the other patients in previous excerpts); rather, she receipts a portion of the justification for the recommendation by objecting to one of the doctor's statements. In excerpt 38, the doctor states his recommendation clearly and then goes on to justify it (portions of this excerpt have been deleted). The patient specifically objects to his claim that there is evidence to support using chemotherapy in women past menopause.

Excerpt 38

198	DR 4	I would recommend that (.) combination
199		chemotherapy be added to the tamoxifen.
200		(1.5)
201		And that it include uh (.) the drug adriamycin.
202		(1.0)
		.
		.
		.
212		Uhm,
213		(1.0)
214		now it's true that combination chemotherapy is not
215		standard therapy. Uhhhm,
216		(1.0)
217		but there are hhh uh some- there is some
218		evidence that uh regimens with adriamycin in them
219		(.) are helpful even in women, uhhh (.) *uh past
220		their menopause.*
221		(0.5)
222	PT 70	Well ih it they did say that it was not helpful.
223		Eh eh as tha- such a small percentage (.) *(was helpful).*

At line 222, the patient objects to the doctor's report that there is evidence in favor of using adriamycin in women past menopause. She accomplishes her objection through a third-party attribution—reporting what "they" said (though "they" never had a full reference) and she produces an emphatic positive (the stressed operator "did"), signaling dispute with an immediately prior utterance (Kleiner & Preston, 1997). She also reproduces the doctor's term ("helpful") though negates it and stresses that negation (line 222). The combination of these elements makes her utterance hearable as a strong objection to the doctor's statement in lines 217–220.

In excerpt 39, the immediate continuation of excerpt 38, the doctor begins his extended turn by offering a qualified agreement with what the patient has just noted, but then counters her objection with an explanation of findings that were presented at a national oncology meeting. Again, the conversational resource of partial agreement allows for consideration of the patient's objection while still moving his own point of view forward.

The doctor's response to the patient's resistance is notable in that it contrasts to Costello's findings in the general medicine clinic where patient objection to recommendations may lead to a reformulation of that recommendation (Costello, 1990, pp. 53–66). In these data, in contrast with Costello's, both strong objections and weak disagreements by patients do not lead to reformulation. Rather, the doctors generally bring out further evidence in favor of their recommendation, as the continuation of this encounter shows.

Excerpt 39

224	DR 4	Uhhhm thee therapies that have been trie:d (.) to
225		date (.) that uh completed data sets that were
226		available uhm fo:r the consensus conference, I
227		agree. Standard therapy, in fact the standard
228		regimen that we give young women (.) is not
229		helpful (in) older women. But uhhhm (.) uh for
230		example, uh there was a (.) paper at the national
231		meetings last year, that was presented in a
232		plenary session.= +now what that means that people
233		thought this was an important enough paper that it
234		was presented at a session where everybody + (.)
235		uh, attended, uhhh looked at (.) uhhhm a standard-
236		compared a standard form of adjuvant therapy, to a
237		standard form with an adriamycin combination added
238		to it. And (.) I think one of the most (. . .)

At the beginning of this turn, the doctor works to delay his expression of agreement with the patient (lines 226–227). The fact that he agrees with her report is buried at the end of his first complete utterance. This seems to be shaped as a qualified or grudging agreement. At line 229, he offers a contrast, introduced with "but," and then provides an example. The use of "for example" is hearable as projecting the evidence to come as just one piece of information out of some larger pool of counterevidence available. The evidence he presents are the findings of a paper presented at the plenary session of a national oncology meeting. Not only does he place stress on the word "plenary" (line 232) but he also attaches a definition and notes how important the paper was ("everybody attended"). The doctor treats the patient as someone in need of the definition, thereby reinforcing, at this critical moment when evidence is being presented, that he is the one with access to specialized knowledge. His role as expert is instantiated through the content of the remark and through the act of defining the term for the patient.

As the talk continues, Patient 70 raises further objections to chemotherapy, again by reporting on a conversation with her other doctor (data not shown). Excerpt 40 begins after the doctor has responded to the patient's query regarding the source of his statistics. And finally, in a strong attempt to convince the patient of the correctness of his recommendation, the doctor raises the stakes by invoking the roles of "doctor" and "patient." He points to the fact that the patient asked for his recommendation. This reminds the patient that his opinion, elicited by her, is something worth listening to. The following excerpt supports the analysis in chapter 3 of the function of gaining a "ticket of entry" into the recommendation early in the encounter. By ticket of entry I meant conversationally achieving the relevance of making a recommendation (by getting a person to ask for advice). The following excerpt demonstrates how the invisible ticket becomes active currency in the effort to persuade the patient to follow a particular course of action. (In this excerpt, HU is the patient's husband.)

Excerpt 40

489	DR 4	Now, [( )
490	HU 70	[*(despite that) my question is*-
491	DR 4	But then uh lemme lemme say this to you though.
492		(2.0)
493	HU 70	.hhhh
494		(1.0)
495	DR 4	This is not cold

496		(1.0)
497		uh science here. Okay? The-you're a patient and
498		I'm a doctor.
499	PT 70	m-hm.
500	DR 4	Uh you asked me what I would recommend to you.=
501	PT 70	=That's right.
502	DR 4	Okay. Uhhhh if 5 years from now, all the studies
503		are in on postoperative adjuvant therapy, and
504		adriamycin clearly is effective
505		(2.0)
506		then it then it's too late for you to get
507		adriamycin.
508		(2.0)

In lines 497–498, the doctor casts them each in a role, thereby conferring certain rights and responsibilities that we attribute to those categories (see Sacks, 1972, on linking categories and activities). Not only does the doctor invoke those particular roles, but he also points to the patient's request for a recommendation. It is important to note here that, as discussed in chapter 3, there is conversational work at the outset of these clinic visits to license the doctor as a legitimate advice-giver, which I argued allows the doctor to gain entry into the task of making a recommendation. Here is a clear example of the doctor using the patient's request for assistance as a resource to remind the patient that he is doing the job she asked him to do. It is clear here that the doctor is making a vigorous effort at convincing the patient of the correctness and even farsightedness of his recommendation. At lines 506–507 he mentions that 5 years from now it will be "too late" for her to profit from what may, in fact, be the best current treatment available. Despite this effort, Doctor 4 does not persuade Patient 70 and she does not ultimately choose the treatment he recommends.

Each of these cases demonstrates that patients are active participants in constructing their understanding of the medical situation. As that understanding emerges, the doctors respond to patients by tempering their optimism or by diminishing their pessimism. Even in the unproblematic case, where the patient easily accepts the recommendation for chemotherapy, the doctor provides both the negative and positive aspects of the treatment she is recommending. Throughout all these examples, and through the rest of the data, doctors are careful to balance the uncertainty of cure with the need to pursue some type of adjuvant therapy. Patients are treated as having the job of deciding what is best for their particular case. We have also seen how at least one doctor invokes his role as doctor to remind the resistant patient that she asked for his assistance and that his recommendation is not only worth considering but also the best course of action.

5.3 Closing the Encounter

Once the doctor and patient have gone through the recommendation and the justification for it and have moved through the objections and concerns, the encounter must be brought to an end. This is accomplished in a variety of ways. In this section I characterize the form and content of the major categories of closing types and then provide a few representative examples.

For the most part, the closings are not critical in the sense that any decisions are made at that point. In other words, it is not as though after the long discussion the patient says, "Okay, doctor. I'm ready for treatment." On the contrary, most patients leave the clinic with the doctor's instruction to "think about" what they have discussed and with the understanding that they can talk on the phone or at another office visit. This is sometimes because the doctor does not have all the information necessary to make a final and firm recommendation—some additional blood test or pathology report is awaited, or the doctor wishes to discuss the case further with colleagues and get back to the patient with a final recommendation. Or, this can simply be the doctor's way of acknowledging that the patient has not spoken in favor of treatment and needs to take some more time to consider the options. In very few cases ($n = 5$ out of 22) the closing of the visit entails discussing the details of getting the treatment started. The majority of closing sections, however, are handled as endings to an encounter that will likely continue at a later date.

From a formal standpoint, closings are initiated by both patients and doctors; either one may open up the ending of the visit. Patients or their co-present friends or family may initiate the closing by mentioning the timeline for a decision. This type of arrangement-making topic is a common mechanism for initiating the closing of ordinary conversation (Schegloff & Sacks, 1973). The following is an example of the patient initiating the closing sequence.

In excerpt 41, the patient and husband have been talking on the topic of the patient's surgical incision. This is not relevant to their previous phase 5 discussion regarding the recommendation, though it is not necessarily "close implicative" either. The actual preclosing begins at line 715.

Excerpt 41

711	HU 97	It was big for job these nurses they were fightin [it.
713	PT 97	[But uhm,
714	HU 97	*I'll tell ya.*
715	PT 97	So we have the weekend to decide. .hhhh
716	DR 4	Right. And uh give me a buzz. Uhm, you got my
717		number?
718	HU 97	Sure do. heh heh heh heh .hhh
719	DR 4	And uh- we had a heck of a time getting you
720		back to you. Were you all away.
721	PT 97	We were. We were sorry about that.
722	DR 4	Oh Okay. We were- I was worried. I thought,
723	HU 97	No.
724	DR 4	*my goodness, something happened er [somethin.*
725	HU	[No. No.

At line 715, the patient initiates the closing by doing "arrangement making"—here by clarifying the timeline for coming to a decision. The doctor responds by requesting that they call him to notify him of the decision (line 716). The talk then continues (lines 719–725) on the topic of the patient's whereabouts prior to the current visit. This talk regarding the patient's whereabouts eventually changes to the topic of the patient's habit of vacationing by the ocean, at which point the doctor mentions that she could get her treatments where she will be vacationing (data not shown). The husband and wife discuss that topic briefly and finally the doctor inserts his commentary into the discussion as shown in line 762 next.

Excerpt 42

762	DR 4	You decide. That's a secondary issue.
763	HU 97	Yeah.
764	DR 4	Give me a buzz on Monday.
765	HU 97	Okay. Doc.
766	PT 97	Okey dokey.
767	HU 97	Thank you again.

The doctor's invitation again for them to call him (line 764) is a commonly used preclosing move by these doctors. This time, the preclosing initiates a final close to the visit (lines 765–767).

Patients may also open up the closing of the clinic visit by asking for the doctor's phone number. The next excerpt provides an example of this—as well as the close-implicative move by the patient to ask for the return of some item in her medical file (a mammogram or pathology slide) that she brought with her. Sometimes, patients simply initiate a "thank you" sequence which initiates the closing. All of these preclosing elements are present in excerpt 45. These elements are indexed as request for phone number (A), request for return of medical record (B), thanking (C), and making arrangements (D).

Excerpt 43

848	HU 83		Uhhhm,
849			(2.5)
850		A→	Is there a (.) telephone number where we can-
851	DR 4		[phone number].
852	HU 83	B→	Okay. And are you through with those
853			mammograms, er
854	DR 4		Yeah.
			.
			.
			.
873	PT 83	C→	/Well thank you do:cto:r./ Appreciate your-
874	DR 4		You're welcome.
875	PT 83		Help. Heh heh
876	DR 4	D→	Look forward to hearing from ya. One way or
877			another.
878	PT 83		Okay [ay.
879	HU 83		[You'll hear.
880	PT 83		We'll let you know.

The final preclosing initiator is offered by the doctor as he mentions arrangements (D).

Doctors may open up the end of the visit by asking the patient if she has any further questions or by simply extending the invitation that the patient call if she has any questions. Doctors also propose that the patient "think about" the treatment options and that a further discussion will take place at a later time.

Excerpt 44

698	DR 5	I think you can probably get through the treatment
699		without too much trouble. Uhh and that's, that's
700		why I feel we ought to use both. But, uhm, I want
701		you to think about it, and we'll make the final
702		decision next week.
703	PT 28	Okay.
704	DR 5	Okay?
705	PT 28	All right.
706	DR 5	Okay. We'll have time to talk more and answer
707		more questions, Okay?
708	PT 28	All right.

Here the doctor reiterates his recommendation (line 700) and then invites the patient to think about that option. There is no pressure on the patient to make her choice immediately. The doctor couches the decision to be made as a joint effort (line 701). The patient receipts the proposed timeline without further question and the doctor offers the final element of the preclosing at line 706.

Clearly, these visits are treated as open-ended sessions in which there is no expectation for an on-the-spot decision. Though doctors generally offer a preclosing element, it is presented in such a way as to indicate that there will be opportunities for further discussions. The visit is closed, but the consultation may continue.

5.4 Conclusion

This chapter looked at how oncologists in these data initially justify the upcoming recommendation for adjuvant therapy. Part of the patient's job is to come to understand the complex medical information being presented in order to choose whether or not to pursue further treatment. To exemplify this process, the excerpts illustrated moments in which patients display their understanding or raise concerns about the efficacy of the proposed treatment for their particular case. Part of the doctor's job is to convey what he or she thinks is in the patient's best interest, without making any guarantees. In this regard, in these excerpts, doctors handled the patient's response to the justification and associated recommendation. In contrast to Costello's findings, the doctors in the current data are not likely to retreat from their recommendations; rather they attempt to fortify the recommendation by bringing to bear further evidence and by invoking their role as an expert.

The oncologists in these data are "up front" about not guaranteeing adjuvant therapy, yet they are firm in countering any patient objection to it. In the process of agreeing with patient concerns and replying to questions, the doctors present themselves as honest and knowledgeable members of their profession. This combination must be, for most patients, a compelling set of traits which make the advice offered seem worth taking.

In closing the encounter, whether patient or doctor initiated, the door is nearly always left open to allow the patient room to further consider the information she has heard and to contact the doctor with any questions. The oncologists close these sessions by presenting themselves as resources for the patient to draw on as needed. This visit is not treated as the final episode in this doctor-patient relationship but as just one more step in the patient's process of coming to understand the complexity of her medical situation.

6

Conclusion

In a filmed interview for a PBS series on the development of human language, Chomsky (1995) remarks:

> The very beginnings of science are always the capacity to be able to be amazed by apparently simple things. For example, if you assume that an apple falls to the ground because that's its natural place—so it's uninteresting—[then] you have no science. If you begin to ask yourself "why does the apple fall to the ground and not rise to the sky;" if you allow yourself to be puzzled by that simple fact, well then you find you have a rather serious question before you. And science begins.

The current research does not pretend to match the contribution to science implied in Chomsky's observation, but this investigation has taken a naive and open position that there is nothing "natural" about the roles of doctor and patient in these medical settings. And there is nothing "natural" about a patient taking a doctor's advice. Instead, I have taken those two observations as researchable phenomena, as categories of action that can be analyzed in terms of participants' language behavior.

If, as some say, talk is an artifact of predetermined roles or social structural position, then the agency of interactants is overlooked in a world where "[b]elief systems grapple with each other in a struggle for control . . . [where] participants could disappear and their beliefs would continue to struggle" (Gill, 1995, p. 25). It may feel awkward to make the conceptual leap to a place where we talk our world into being, where interaction constructs our roles from moment to moment, but to do so expands the horizon for understanding social action and interaction. The early breaching experiments by Garfinkel demonstrated that people orient to rules that are constitutive of social action but are, at the same time, so taken for granted as to seem "only natural." And therein lies an enormous opportunity: to research what we take for granted; by subjecting our commonsense notions to close scrutiny we come to learn how the world is constructed through talk-in-interaction.

Taking that opportunity, this study began with an exercise in audiotape archaeology (see chapter 2) as an attempt to hear the participants' verbal behavior as naively as possible. I knew very little about the interactants and never felt the need to know more — their displayed orientations to one another revealed so much. Assumptions about the relative status of oncologists and patients did not help me to understand their activities; the participants themselves revealed what was relevant for them. In this way I was able to note how patients and doctors cooperate in the creation and maintenance of their roles, and how recommendations for cancer treatment are delivered and received as part of a broader medical interaction.

Language researchers in schools, businesses, and other institutional settings may find the approach taken in this book to be useful for illuminating aspects of "role" that are simply taken for granted in those settings. By doing so, new understanding will be gained about the structure of talk-in-interaction and its function as a fine-grained organizer of the setting and participants. It may be more instructive and productive to look at role as a *resource* in interaction than as a predetermined set of beliefs, rights, and responsibilities.

The current research represents the first attempt to fully describe and analyze the ways in which doctors and patients interact through language to create a forum in which recommendations for cancer treatment are given and received. This is a baseline study of a very complex interactional setting and as such does not exhaust the possible actions or orientations that participants are taking in these encounters. Thus any findings should be read as provisional and subject to further study. This investigation offers one way to characterize one set of medical encounters and provides a preliminary sketch of the activities integral to the overall accomplishment of these oncology visits. Whether or not these findings are generalizable to other oncology clinics is an empirical matter, to be taken up in future studies.

6.1 Review of Findings

In the introduction to this book I mentioned two observations that were not particularly startling: (1) that a substantial portion of the treatment recommendation visit is devoted to topics aside from explicit discussion of the recommendation, and (2) that there is a sense throughout the encounter that doctors are attempting to persuade patients to take a particular course of action. The first observation gave rise to the research question: What is all this talk accomplishing? The second led me to wonder: Why *do* we take advice from other people? These rather broad questions have led to some important conclusions about what the talk in these interactions is doing and how that work is getting done. To a great extent, actions that were not explicitly "doing recommending" were working to create and maintain the occasion as appropriate for advice-giving: The allocation of turns and turn types, verbal management of the medical agenda, displays of access to knowledge, resistance to or engagement with patient troubles-talk—all these were doing the work necessary for constructing the occasion as one in which medical recommendations or advice-giving became a legitimate activity.

Until recently, the asymmetrical roles of doctor and patient have simply been seen as a given in the medical setting: Doctors are powerful, knowledgeable, and expert, patients are not; therefore, doctors control the situation. But that kind of explanation leaves completely unanalyzed the mechanics of how power or control is achieved through talk and how expertise is a resource to be strategically deployed by both doctors and patients. Findings from this research, along with studies by ten Have (1991), Heath (1992), Gill (1995), and Barton (1996), confirm that "doctors and patients sustain *who they are* through *what they do*. . . ." (Gill, 1995, p.196), where the "what" refers to conversational mechanisms that are oriented to by the interactants in the moments of their ongoing talk. This approach to understanding medical interaction provides analytic backbone to otherwise taken-for-granted phenomena.

In the current study, management of the agenda in the ways outlined in chapters 3 and 4 provides a new perspective on how it is that asymmetrical control of medical encounters is achieved. As ten Have (1991) points out, discourse approaches to asymmetry have treated this aspect of doctor-patient communication from the narrow point of view of doctors' questioning behavior. In this study, rather than simply assuming the doctor had control and leaving that unanalyzed, we looked at the mechanics of control across a range of activities, not just episodes of questioning. The "how" question was answered here in terms of specific conversational strategies such as uncontested doctor-initiated adjacency pairs; that is, patients passing the opportunity to take a turn during the medical information phase of the visit; topic shifts, which reassert the medical agenda; doctor turns, which are constructed to display dispreference for patient questions at particular points in the encounter; and turn continuing, which sequentially deletes patient contributions.

In terms of expertise, these encounters are structured such that knowledge will be shared—but only at the appropriate time. The "appropriateness" is not simply a matter of externally imposed formal constraints on the interaction; it is constitutive of the role that the oncologist has as gatekeeper and as such instantiates his or her expertise in the setting. Doctors present themselves as experts by displaying access to information and by controlling the flow of that information. The latter is accomplished through some of the same conversational mechanisms mentioned earlier (e.g., dispreference for patient questions, topic shifts) as well as through the use of rhetorical questions which set up the relevance of upcoming information. These tend to appear in extended turns, where the doctor is continuing an explanation. Ainsworth-Vaughn (1994) refers to the use of rhetorical questions in this position as the doctor adopting the patient's voice to display understanding of the patient's likely questions (pp. 200–201). However one chooses to interpret the use of rhetorical questions in extended turns, it is clear that they function to introduce new information and, when treated as rhetorical by the co-participant, retain the floor for the speaker in progress, usually the doctor (as expert) in these data.

For their part, patients appeal to the doctor as someone who *is* expert and capable of providing information about their medical status. They achieve this not only by asking the doctor questions about their health and treatment options but also by *not* pursuing topics that the doctor has treated in some way as currently irrelevant or "out of order" (chapter 3).

These interactions also include important work to establish and maintain the stance and face of the patients, who present themselves as educable, reasonable, and flexible persons (chapter 4). This is accomplished cooperatively: by the patients' presentation of their preparedness (e.g., through mention of prior reading) and by doctors who treat that preparedness as noteworthy. This shared effort casts the patient as an informed and informable advice-seeker.

The talk and actions briefly reviewed thus far are about displaying roles of expert/novice, establishing knowledgeability, and creating a context for the transfer of new information. All these factors may contribute to motivating the patient to follow the doctor's recommendation, though the current investigation does not allow us to speculate too widely in that direction.

Finally, the work of the medical recommendation itself is accomplished through the talk. As discussed in chapter 5, patients display their understanding of the complex medical information being presented to them by offering assessments of the information they have been hearing. They may appeal to third parties to shore up reports or claims that they are making in opposition to the doctor's point of view. For their part, doctors work to convey what is in the patient's best interest, without making any guarantees. Specifically, they temper patient assessments through delayed agreements and disagreements and use rhetorical questions and historical accounts to move their argument for treatment forward.

All these accomplishments, whether the cooperative construction of an asymmetrical power relationship, the establishment of expertise, or the rendering and reception of the recommendation are conversational achievements. Specific conversational mechanisms work to establish an appropriate forum for giving and receiving expert advice as well as to shape the discussion of a recommended treatment option.

6.2 Future Research

By amplifying the scope of the study to include all the phases that surround "the recommendation," I hope to have set the stage for future investigations to consider in detail the phase in which the recommendation itself resides. Though I might have restricted myself to that penultimate phase of the oncology visit, it was apparent that I had to first provide a detailed description of the whole visit so that eventually its parts could be examined and understood for their contribution to the recommendation phase. As with any study of this scope, the findings have prompted new confidence and new questions.

Maynard's work on the co-implication of patients in the delivery of bad news (Maynard, 1991a, 1991b, 1992), Heritage and Sefi's treatment of the ticket-of-entry problem among home health visitors (Heritage & Sefi, 1992), and my own analysis of how the oncologists in these data make relevant in phase 2 the advice to come in phase 5 all point to similar patterns of interaction across institutional settings. This attests to the strength of conversation analysis for uncovering significant and recurrent actions accomplished through talk. Further refinement of these observations in other institutional and ordinary settings will yield deeper insight into how participants interact to accomplish the day-to-day work of talking their personal and institutional roles into being. This may also lead to a better understanding of how to work more successfully with clients in institutional settings.

The shape of the uninterrupted and extended patient turns in phase 2 of the medical encounters studied here is in sharp contrast to findings from investigations of general medical visits. What it means to be a patient in this oncology setting seems to be very different from what it means to be some other kind of patient. This finding requires refinement through analyses of talk in other oncology clinics as this may be a characteristic of the particular setting in which the data were collected.

The current investigation also finds that the recommendation in an oncology setting is not as easily negotiable as Costello (1990) found it to be in the general medical setting. In these data, patients can be quite staunch in their resistance to a recommendation. With this knowledge, we can now further investigate the problem of age bias in cancer treatment and determine, perhaps more precisely, what the sources of that bias are. Though studies have typically focused on the physicians' contribution to differential treatment of older and younger patients (see chapter 1, in this volume), we begin to see more clearly in this research that patient resistance to treatment and how that resistance is handled may also play a role in the outcome measure of "treatment choice." How oncologists respond to patient resistance, what steps they take (or not) to further their arguments for or against treatment, can only be revealed by doing detailed analysis of actual conversations in the clinic. Retrospective approaches and vignette approaches may never capture these crucial moments of interaction. Quantitative analyses may not prove fruitful until we have had a close look at other cancer recommendation visits and can confidently identify recurrent patterns of conversational activity.

In this study, the recommendation portion of the visit was seen to be a complex phenomenon comprising both a justification and a recommendation. Patients actively questioned the doctor to make sense of the information as it was presented. Also, doctors tempered patient optimism as well as patient pessimism, always seeming to walk a fine line between not making any guarantees and still promoting a particular course of treatment.

The persuasive aspect of the talk, however, needs further investigation.

For example, the distribution of pronoun forms and their function as anchors of alignment with the institution (or not) could be undertaken to better understand the shape of the oncologist's unfolding argument about treatment. The institutional weight of the first-person plural (we) is juxtaposed in these data with the oncologist's personal (I) alignment with some information or advice. This is a rich area of exploration, as is the oncologists' use of the first-person singular pronoun form to animate patient concerns, putting him or herself "in the patient's shoes" at particularly problematic points in the treatment discussions.

This research makes an important contribution to the medical literature on both cancer recommendations and treatment bias, as most investigations have tended to ignore spoken interaction. The seminal work in this field has looked at what the participants (i.e., doctors) would do in hypothetical cases (vignette studies) or what they remembered doing (retrospective studies), but very little work has been done to examine what the participants *actually do.* In this way, I hope this project will be useful to those who wish to better understand the conversational dynamic of oncologist-patient interaction and help them in framing the next generation of questions on the topic.

Because the particular topic of this research is focused on breast cancer treatment, perhaps findings from this investigation will also be consequential for women facing the related, rather daunting medical decisions. Although there are currently no clinical applications for this research, this investigation represents the first step toward more fully understanding the dynamics of the doctor-patient relationship in the oncology setting. Through talk and through action, the participants have artfully and accomplished an intricate pattern of social and medical face-to-face interaction. As the analyst, I have tried to bring the subtle to awareness, to reveal parts of the pattern and to make sense of what all their talk is doing.

Appendix A

Patient Information

Table A.1 Demographic Characteristics

Patient	Marital Status	Race	Age	Educ	Religion	Children
2	1	1	43	3	3	6
26	1	1	36	4	2	4
27	1	1	44	3	3	2
28	2	2	68	3	3	0
30	1	1	41	5	2	2
37	1	1	56	4	3	3
43	1	1	40	5	2	4
44	1	1	65	2	3	3
46	4	2	66	4	3	0
50	1	1	34	5	1	2
53	1	1	22	3	2	0
58	1	1	43	3	2	3
59	1	1	40	5	3	3
60	1	2	33	3	2	1
70	1	1	66	5	1	2
76	1	1	65	5	4	3
83	1	1	53	5	3	2
91	1	1	55	4	2	4
92	1	1	36	4	2	1
96	3	2	73	2	3	3
97	1	1	69	3	2	5
101	Data not available for this patient.					

Note. Variable values are as follows.

Married: 1 = married; 2 = divorced/separated; 3 = never married; 4 = widow.
Race: 1 = White; 2 = Black; 3 = Hispanic; 4 = Asian; 5 = other.
Education: 1 = 0–6 yrs; 2 = 7–11 yrs; 3 = hs grad; 4 = some coll; 5 = coll grad.
Religion: 1 = none; 2 = Catholic; 3 = Protestant; 4 = Jewish; 5 = other.
Children: Number of children.

Table A.2 Medical Characteristics

Pt	Pos Nodes	Menops Status	Tumor Size	Estrog Receptr	Proges Receptr	Prim Treatmt	Stage	Recom	Option Chosen
2	1	2	2	16	98	8	2	2	2
26	2	1	3	0	0	8	3	1	1
27	1	1	1	38	98	7	2	1	1
28	1	2	2	98	98	8	2	8	8
30	1	1	1	59	99	8	2	10	1
37	3	2	3	33	25	8	3	12	8
43	3	1	3	98	27	8	3	17	17
44	1	2	1	98	48	8	2	9	9
46	2	2	1	0	0	8	2	7	7
50	0	1	1	98	98	5	1	0	0
53	0	1	2	19	98	8	2	20	20
58	1	1	1	39	86	8	2	1	1
59	1	1	2	33	43	8	2	1	10
60	0	1	3	0	0	8	3	20	20
70	2	2	2	14	6	8	2	8	9
76	3	2	1	98	98	8	2	8	9
83	1	2	2	98	0	8	2	2	2
91	3	2	2	98	21	8	2	8	7
92	0	1	3	0	0	8	3	1	1
96	0	2	3	0	0	8	1	0	0
97	1	2	1	0	0	8	2	7	7
101	Data not available for this patient.								

Note. Variable values are as follows.
Positive nodes: 0 = none; 1 = 1–3; 2 = 4–9; 3 = 10+.
Menopausal status: 1 = premenopausal; 2 = postmenopausal.
Tumor size: 1 = 2 cm or less; 2 = >2–<5 cms; 3 = 5+ cms.
Estrogen receptor: Test value for tumor receptivity to estrogen.
Progesterone receptor: Test value for tumor receptivity to progesterone.
Primary treatment: 0 = none; 1 = biopsy; 2 = lumpectomy; 3 = lump and node dissection; 4 = simple mastectomy; 5 = simple mastectomy and node dissection; 6 = quadrilateral surgery; 7 = quadrilateral and node dissection; 8 = modified radical mastectomy; 9 = radical mastectomy. (These refer to combinations [or not] of surgical procedure [e.g., biopsy or mastectomy] with axillary node dissection: Lymph nodes in the surrounding tissue are removed to determine if there has been any spread of malignant cells into them.)
Stage: 1 = Stage I; 2 = Stage II; 3 = Stage III. (Extent of disease is staged according to size of tumor and spread of the cancer.)
Recommendation: 0 = no treatment; 1 = CMF; 2 = CMFT; 3 = CMFP; 4 = CMFPT; 5 = CMFVP; 6 = CMFVPT; 7 = CAF; 8 = CAFT; 9 = T only; 10 = premno trial; 11 = postmen trial; 12 = 10 node trial, 13 = node neg trial; 14 = clin tr; 15 = radiation; 16 = no rec; 17 = other; 18 = chemo gen; 19 = NodenegF; 20 = unknown. (Treatment recommended by the oncologist. These treatment options are various combinations of chemotherapeutic agents, hormonal or steroidal agents, radiation, and different options for clinical trials.)
Option chosen: Same values as given in Recommendation.

Appendix B

Transcription Symbols

(based on Jefferson, 1974)

.	Falling, "final" intonation
,	Continuing, "comma" intonation
?	Rising intonation
:	Sound stretch
CAPS	Louder than surrounding talk
* *	Reduced volume between these signs
+ +	Faster speech between these signs
___	(underline) Stressed element
/ /	Speech between these signs is hearable as higher in pitch
☺	"Smiling face" indicates onset of a smile voice in the talk
huh	(or variant heh) Transcription of burst of laughter
.hhh	Audible inbreath
hhh	Audible outbreath
(.)	Untimed "micropause"
(1.0)	Timed pause, represented in seconds
=	Talk that is latched
[	Marks onset of overlap
-	(hyphen) Speaker cuts own speech
( )	Transcriber doubt, utterance indecipherable
((sniff))	Untranscribed sound or transcriber comments
...	(horizontal or vertical ellipses) Lines of text deleted

Notes

Chapter 1. Introduction

1. Most research investigating the apparent age bias in breast cancer treatment has been biomedical and includes studies by Allen, Cox, Manton, & Cohen, 1986; Chu, Diehr, Feigl, Glaefke, Begg, Glicksman, & Ford, 1987; Greenfield, Blanco, Elashoff, & Ganz, 1987; Silliman, Guadagnoli, Weitberg, & Mor, 1989; andYancik, Ries, & Yates, 1989. What this research has found is that given similar disease profiles, younger patients (defined usually as ≤ 65 years old) tend to receive more aggressive treatment than do older ones, particularly in terms of adjuvant chemotherapy for breast cancer.

The assumption underlying most research on age bias is that physician preferences are driving the apparent disparity in cancer treatment. Research suggests that doctors tend not to recommend chemotherapy to older women because of concerns about comorbid conditions, perceived patient frailty, and insufficient data on older women in clinical trials of adjuvant chemotherapy (Satariano, Ragheb, & Dupuis, 1989; Silliman, Balducci, Goodwin, Holmes, Leventhal, 1993). However, Newcomb & Carbone (1993) conclude from their patient retrospection study that patient preferences also affect selection of breast cancer treatments. This finding seems intuitively plausible and requires further investigation, both within the context of the clinic visit and as a longitudinal concern.

2. As Pomerantz and Fehr (1997) point out in their endnote no. 6, analysis of temporal and sequential organization is not a "defining" feature of CA, but it is

what distinguishes CA from other discourse approaches. It is worth noting from a practical standpoint that in working with the data for this study I found it extremely important and useful to anchor myself to the notion of sequence as I came to slowly "unpack" the actions and orientations of the participants.

3. Harvey Sacks (1987) writes, in an essay published posthumously, that "ready observability need not imply banality, and, therefore, silence" (p. 56). He is arguing for the need to "come to terms with" mundane conversational occurrences. He reports the observation that second pair parts are type-related to first pair parts; for example, answers follow questions in particular ways. Though this is a simple observation, by analyzing this observable phenomenon and examining the full range of its contingencies, Sacks reveals something about how talk-in-interaction is organized, and therefore how a "sector of the world" is organized.

Though I do not claim that my observations will bring insights on the level of Harvey Sacks's revelations about social order, I am committed to examining the "totally observable" as a means for understanding a particular sector of the world.

4. From a clinical point of view, physician "expertise" is not all-powerful. Patient compliance with physician recommendations is notoriously difficult to achieve; patients do not simply follow their doctors' advice. Indeed, understanding this problematic area of medical practice has produced a monumental body of literature. In the span of 20 years, nearly 4,000 articles have been produced by "compliance researchers" (Trostle, 1988: 1299).

5. An important contribution of the conversation analytic approach is to refine our understanding of what is an analytically relevant "speech act"—if indeed there is such a thing. It has been shown that it is enormously difficult to simply "pull out" examples of linguistic items which are also interactionally relevant. This is particularly salient in research on questioning in medical encounters.

As West (1984a) points out in an analysis of the distribution of questions for managing misunderstandings, conditionally relevant queries (requests for confirmation, requests for repair, and surprise markers) are more symmetrically distributed than other types of questions in medical interaction. She excluded the class of conditionally relevant queries in her first analysis (West, 1983), realizing that those question-looking things were actually accomplishing something quite different from other question-like entities. And Frankel (1983) notes how nonmedical questions are used to direct the visual attention of the pediatric patient away from the work of the physician's hands and toward the task of conversing (p. 44).

Without this kind of attention to interactional relevance, there is a danger of lumping all question-like things together, and one would miss important insight into mechanisms for managing misunderstandings on the one hand (West, 1984a) or managing patient visual attention on the other (Frankel, 1983). The analytic intractability of "questions" in medical encounters is also discussed in the work by ten Have (1991) in his treatment of patient formulation of their "ignorance" (as patients) as a covert information-seeking strategy.

In brief, setting limits on the category "question"—an object often excised from naturally occurring conversation and treated as countable in studies of medical interaction—has been shown to be a highly problematic linguistic construct. The evidence suggests that other speech act categories may be equally impervious to analytic separation from their natural habitat of talk-in-interaction.

6. Steele et al. (1990) is actually a qualitative study of conversational strategies used by physicians to assess patient adherence to treatment (in this case, the use of antihypertensive medication). The article presents excerpts of transcribed talk to exemplify three categories of adherence-monitoring practices. Steele then assesses the effectiveness of those approaches by comparing pre-visit patient responses to interview questions about adherence to physician success at eliciting self-reports about adherence during the clinic visit. I include the study by Steele et al. here because it is primarily concerned with patient adherence, even though qualitative methodology is not typical of the other studies cited as being "sociomedical."

7. Though some discourse studies introduce distributional analysis of "speech acts" into their work (such as relative proportions of questions or directives delivered by physicians and patients) and thus might be viewed as quantitative, they also recognize the importance of treating the interaction as an ongoing discourse and usually provide examples of transcribed talk to support their analysis. In fact, discourse studies often present themselves as reactions against, and improvements upon, the more abstract, quantitative studies in the sociomedical tradition.

Chapter 3. Phased Organization of the Adjuvant Therapy Visit

1. The following is a brief explanation of the four cases in which the patient's perspective is not specifically elicited by the doctor. In the first, the doctor clearly states that he has recently spoken on the phone with the patient. They begin their clinic visit with an immediate discussion of phase 4 topics.

PT 37 and DR 4

DR 4 What I'm recommending? is that we not let nature take its
course.=That we try to improve the odds. Now I want to make it
very clear to you Ms. [B] cuz you've made this clear to me over
the phone, [continues]

In the second case, the audio recording picks up well after the initiation of the visit and it is impossible to know if the doctor had asked the patient about her understanding of her current medical condition. Nonetheless, the doctor does raise information about lymph node status.

In the two other cases, the doctor asked how the patient was "feeling" in general without specific reference to "where she stands" at the moment or specifically what brought her to the oncology clinic that day. The doctor provides his own summary of the patient's current status which the patient ratifies. The following excerpt is an example:

PT 28 and DR 5

1	PT 28	I keep a close watch on my eyes.
2	DR 5	Good. good.
3		(3.5)
4		Okay. Um? let's talk about your- the the breast cancer.
5	PT 28	[mm
6	DR 5	[Um,
7		(3.5)
8		Doctor M (.) of course has removed the breast. And
9		the breast did <u>not</u> have any residual cells in it.
10	PT 28	[mm
11	DR 5	[okay?
12	PT 28	mm.
13	DR 5	um but we <u>do</u> have some concern because [*of the lymph*
14		*nodes removed*] three of them had some cancer cells in them.

Chapter 4. Discourse Identities: Establishing Participant Roles as Doctor and Patient

1. The patient's laughter after her announcement "that's all I have to say" can be seen as troubles resistant (Jefferson, 1984). She displays herself as managing in the face of some difficulty. It is hard to know here whether the difficulty she is managing is the fact that she had no insurance or that she has just told the doctor she won't speak further on the issue. The fact that the doctor does not take up the laughter but simply responds to the content of her utterance is indicative that he is in a troubles-receptive stance (Jefferson, 1984). This shows that he is not taking the situation lightly and shows alignment with her grievance even though she herself is trying to downplay it.

2. Progesterone and estrogen receptors are indicators of the chemical composition of the tumor. These test values are prognostic factors in that hormonal receptivity can indicate the speed at which the tumor may have grown/is growing. The decision whether or not to treat breast cancer with tamoxifan (an antiestrogen) is based, to some extent, on the hormonal composition of the tumor.

3. When I say that the concerns are addressed as they are raised, this does not necessarily mean that there is an answer for the patient. In other words, the doctor may immediately address the question with an answer, though the answer may simply be an admission that knowledge about causation is still rather thin.

References

Ainsworth-Vaughn, N. (1992). Topic transitions in physician-patient interviews: Power, gender, and discourse change. *Language in Society, 21*, 409-426.

Ainsworth-Vaughn, N. (1994). Is that a rhetorical question? Ambiguity and power in medical discourse. *Journal of Linguistic Anthropology, 4*(2), 194–214.

Allen, C., Cox, E. B., & Manton, K. G., & Cohen, H. J. (1986). Breast cancer in the elderly: Current patterns. *Journal of the American Geriatric Society, 34*, 637–642.

Amir, M. (1987). Considerations guiding physicians when informing cancer patients. *Social Science and Medicine, 24*(9), 741–748.

Atkinson, J. M., & Drew, P. (1979). *Order in court: The organization of verbal interaction in judicial settings*. London: Macmillan.

Barton, E. L. (1996). Negotiating expertise in discourses of disability. *Text, 16*(3), 299–322.

Beckman, H. B., & Frankel, R. M. (1984). The effect of physician behavior on the collection of data. *Annals of Internal Medicine, 101*, 692–696.

Bourhis, R. Y., Roth, S., & MacQueen, G. (1989). Communication in the hospital setting: A survey of medical and everyday language use amongst patients, nurses and doctors. *Social Science and Medicine, 28*(4), 339–346.

Buller, M. K., & Buller, D. B. (1987). Physicians' communication style and patient satisfaction. *Journal of Health and Social Behavior, 28*, 375–388.

Byrne, P. S., & Long, B. E. L. (1976). *Doctors talking to patients: A study of the verbal behaviors of doctors in the consultation.* London: HMSO.

Chomsky, N. (1995). Discovering the human language: "Colorless green ideas." In G. Searchinger (Producer), *The human language series—Part I.* New York: Equinox Films.

Chu, J., Diehr, P., Feigl, P., Glaefke, G., Begg, C., Glicksman, A., & Ford, L. (1987). The effect of age on the care of women with breast cancer in community hospitals. *Journal of Gerontology, 42,* 185–190.

Cicourel, A. V. (1974). *Cognitive sociology.* New York: Free Press.

Cicourel, A. V. (1981). Language and medicine. In C. A. Ferguson & S. Brice Heath (Eds.), *Language in the USA*. Cambridge: Cambridge University Press.

Cicourel, A. V. (1983). Hearing is not believing: Language and the structure of belief in medical communication. In S. Fisher & A. Dundas Todd (Eds.), *The social organization of doctor-patient communication* (pp. 221–239). Washington, DC: Center for Applied Linguistics.

Cicourel, A. V. (1992). The interpenetration of communicative contexts: Examples from medical encounters. In A. Duranti & C. Goodwin (Eds.), *Rethinking context: Language as an interactive phenomenon* (pp. 291–310). Cambridge: Cambridge University Press.

Clayman, S. E. (1988). Displaying neutrality in television news interviews. *Social Problems, 35*(4), 474–492.

Clayman, S. E. (1992). Footing in the achievement of neutrality: The case of news-interview discourse. In P. Drew & J. Heritage (Eds.), *Talk at work: Interaction in institutional settings* (pp. 163–198). Cambridge: Cambridge University Press.

Collins, G. E. (1955) Do we really advise the patient? *Journal of the Florida Medical Association, 42*(2), 111–115.

Costello, B. (1990). The delivery and receipt of recommendations in the doctor-patient encounter. Unpublished M.A. thesis, University of Wisconsin-Madison.

Davis, M. S. (1968). Variations in patients' compliance with doctors' advice: An empirical analysis of patterns of communication. *American Journal of Public Health, 58*(2), 274–288.

Drew, P., & Heritage, J. (1992). Analyzing talk at work: An introduction. In P. Drew & J. Heritage (Eds.), *Talk at work: Interaction in institutional settings* (pp. 3–65). Cambridge: Cambridge University Press.

Duranti A., & Goodwin, C. (1992). *Rethinking context: Language as an interactive phenomenon.* Cambridge: Cambridge University Press.

Fisher, S. (1982). The decision making context: How doctor and patient communicate. In R. J. Di Pietro (Ed.), *Linguistics and the professions* (pp. 51–81). Norwood, NJ: Ablex.

Fisher, S. (1983). Doctor talk/patient talk: How treatment decisions are negotiated in doctor-patient communication. In S. Fisher & A. Dundas Todd (Eds.), *The social organization of doctor-patient communication* (pp. 135–157). Washington, DC: Center for Applied Linguistics.

Fisher, S. (1984). Institutional authority and the structure of discourse. *Discourse Processes, 7*, 201–224.

Ford, C. E., Fox, B., & Thompson, S. A. (1996). Practices in the construction of turns: The "TCU" revisited. *Pragmatics, 6*(3), 427–454.

Ford, C. E., & Thompson, S. A. (1996). Interactional units in conversation: Syntactic, intonational, and pragmatic resources for the management of turns. In E. Ochs, E. A. Schegloff, & S. A. Thompson (Eds.), *Interaction and grammar* (pp. 134–184). Cambridge: Cambridge University Press.

Ford, S., Fallowfield, L., & Lewis, S. (1996). Doctor-patient interactions in oncology. *Social Science and Medicine, 42*(11), 1511–1519.

Frankel, R. M. (1983). The laying on of hands: Aspects of the organization of gaze, touch, and talk in a medical encounter. In S. Fisher & A. Dundas Todd (Eds.), *The social organization of doctor-patient communication* (pp. 19–54). Washington, DC: Center for Applied Linguistics.

Frankel, R. M. (1984). From sentence to sequence: Understanding the medical encounter through microinteractional analysis. *Discourse Processes, 7*, 135–170.

Frankel, R. M. (1989). Talking in interviews: A dispreference for patient initiated questions in physician-patient encounters. In G. Psathas (Ed.), *Interaction competence: Studies in ethnomethodology and conversation analysis, No. 1* (pp. 231–262). Lanham, MD: University Press of America.

Garfinkel, H. (1967). *Studies in ethnomethodology*. Englewood Cliffs, NJ: Prentice Hall.

Garfinkel, H., & Sacks, H. (1970). On formal structures of practical actions. In J. C. McKinney & E. A. Tiryakian (Eds.), *Theoretical sociology* (pp. 338–366). New York: Appleton-Century-Crofts.

Gill, V. T. (1995). The organization of patients' explanations and doctors' responses in clinical interaction. Unpublished Ph.D. dissertation, University of Wisconsin-Madison.

Greenfield, S., Blanco, D. M., & Elashoff, R. M., & Ganz, P.A. (1987). Patterns of care related to age of breast cancer patients. *Journal of the American Medical Association, 257*, 2766–2770.

Hadlow, J., & Pitts, M. (1991). The understanding of common health terms by doctors, nurses and patients. *Social Science and Medicine, 32*(2), 193–196.

Halkowski, T. (1990) "Role" as an interactional device. *Social Problems, 37*(4), 564–577.

Hall, J. A., Roter, D. L., & Katz, N. R. (1988). Meta-analysis of correlates of provider behavior in medical encounters. *Medical Care, 26*(7), 657–673.

Heath, C. (1992). The delivery and reception of diagnosis in the general-practice consultation. In P. Drew & J. Heritage (Eds.), *Talk at work: Interaction in institutional settings* (pp. 235–267). Cambridge: Cambridge University Press.

Heritage, J. (1984). *Garfinkel and ethnomethodology*. Cambridge: Polity Press.

Heritage, J., & Roth, A. L. (1995). Grammar and institution: Questions and questioning in the broadcast news interview. *Research on Language and Social Interaction, 28*(1), 1–60.

Heritage, J., & Sefi, S. (1992). Dilemmas of advice: Aspects of the delivery and reception of advice in interactions between health visitors and first-time mothers. In P. Drew & J. Heritage (Eds.), *Talk at work: Interaction in institutional settings* (pp. 359–417). Cambridge: Cambridge University Press.

Heritage, J., & Sorjonen, M. (1994). Constituting and maintaining activities across sequences: *And*-prefacing as a feature of question design. *Language in Society, 23,* 1–29.

Jefferson, G. (1974). Error correction as an interactional resource. *Language in Society, 2,* 191–199.

Jefferson, G. (1984a). On stepwise transition from talk about a trouble to inappropriately next-positioned matters. In J. M. Atkinson & J. Heritage (Eds.), *Structures of social action: Studies in conversation analysis* (pp. 191–222). Cambridge: Cambridge University Press.

Jefferson, G. (1984b). On the organization of laughter in talk about troubles. In J. M. Atkinson & J. Heritage (Eds.), *Structures of social action: Studies in conversation analysis* (pp. 347–369). Cambridge: Cambridge University Press.

Jefferson, G., & Lee, J. R. E. (1992). The rejection of advice: Managing the problematic convergence of a "troubles-telling" and a "service encounter." In P. Drew & J. Heritage (Eds.), *Talk at work: Interaction in institutional settings* (pp. 521–548). Cambridge: Cambridge University Press.

Jefferson, G., Sacks, H., & Schegloff, E. (1987). Notes on laughter in the pursuit of intimacy. In G. Button & J. R. E. Lee (Eds.), *Talk and social organization* (pp. 152–205). Clevedon, England: Multilingual Matters.

Kleiner, B., & Preston, D. R. (1997). Discourse disputes: How come you do do like you do? *Folia Linguistica, 31*(1/2), 105–131.

Korsch, B. M., & Negrete, V. F. (1972). Doctor-patient communication. *Scientific American, 227*, 66.

Labov, W., & Fanshell, D. (1977). *Therapeutic discourse: Psychotherapy as conversation.* New York: Academic Press.

Laine, C., & Davidoff, F. (1996). Patient-centered medicine: A professional evaluation. *Journal of the American Medical Association, 275*(2), 152–156.

Levinson, S. C. (1983). *Pragmatics.* Cambridge: Cambridge University Press.

Liberati, A., Apolone, G., Nicolucci, A., Confalonieri, C., Fossati, R., Grilli, R., Torri, V., Mosconi, P., & Alexanian, A. (1990). The role of attitudes, beliefs, and personal characteristics of Italian physicians in the surgical treatment of breast cancer. *American Journal of Public Health, 81,* 38–42.

Local, J. (1992). Continuing and restarting. In P. Auer & A. DiLuzio (Eds.), *The contextualization of language* (pp. 273–296). Amsterdam: John Benjamins.

Maynard, D. (1991a). Bearing bad news in clinical settings. In B. Dervin & M. J. Voight (Eds.), *Progress in communication sciences* (pp. 143–172). Norwood, NJ: Ablex.

Maynard, D. (1991b). The perspective-display series and the delivery and receipt of diagnostic news. In D. Boden & D. H. Zimmerman (Eds.), *Talk and social structure: Studies in ethnomethodology and conversation analysis* (pp. 164–192). Cambridge, MA: Polity Press.

Maynard, D. (1992). On clinicians co-implicating recipients' perspective in delivery of diagnostic news. In P. Drew & J. Heritage (Eds.), *Talk at work: Interaction in institutional settings* (pp. 331–358). Cambridge: Cambridge University Press.

McKinlay, J. B. (1975). Who is really ignorant—physician or patient? *Journal of Health and Social Behavior, 164*(1), 3–11.

Mishler, E. (1984). *The discourse of medicine: Dialectics of medical interviews.* Norwood, NJ: Ablex.

Moerman, M. (1988). *Talking culture: Ethnography and conversation analysis.* Philadelphia: University of Pennsylvania Press.

Newcomb, P. A., & Carbone, P. (1993). Cancer treatment and age: Patient perspectives. *Journal of the National Cancer Institute, 85*(19), 1580–1584.

Ochs, E. (1979). Transcription as theory. In E. Ochs & B. B. Schiefflin (Eds.), *Developmental pragmatics* (pp. 43–72). New York: Academic Press.

Ong, L. M. L., DeHaes, J. C. J. M., Hoos, A. M., & Lammes, F. B. (1995). Doctor-patient communication: A review of the literature. *Social Science and Medicine, 40*(7), 903–918.

Phillips, D. (1996). Medical professional dominance and client dissatisfaction. *Social Science and Medicine, 42*(10), 1419–1425.

Pomerantz, A. (1984). Agreeing and disagreeing with assessments: Some features of preferred/dispreferred turn shapes. In J. M. Atkinson & J. Heritage (Eds.), *Structures of social action: Studies in conversation analysis* (pp. 57–101). Cambridge: Cambridge University Press.

Pomerantz, A. (1988). Offering a candidate answer: An information seeking strategy. *Communication Monographs, 55,* 360–373.

Pomerantz, A., & Fehr, B. J. (1997). Conversation analysis: An approach to the study of social action as sense making. In T. A. Van Dijk (Ed.), *Discourse as social interaction* (pp. 64–91). London: Sage.

Psathas, G. (1995). *ConversationAnalysis: The Study ofTalk-in-Interaction.* Thousand Oaks, CA: Sage.

Roter, D., & Frankel, F. (1992). Quantitative and qualitative approaches to the evaluation of the medical dialogue. *Social Science and Medicine, 34*(10), 1097–1103.

Roter, D. L., & Hall, J. A. (1992). *Doctors talking with patients/Patients talking with doctors: Improving communication in medical visits.* Westport, CT: Auburn House.

Roter, D. L., Hall, J. A., & Katz, N. R. (1988). Patient-physician communication: A descriptive summary of the literature. *Patient Education and Counseling, 12,* 99–119.

Sacks, H. (1972). On the analyzability of stories by children. In J. Gumperz & D. Hymes (Eds.), *Directions in sociolinguistics* (pp. 325–345). New York: Holt,

Rinehart & Winston.

Sacks, H. (1984). Notes on methodology. In J. M. Atkinson & J. Heritage (Eds.), *Structures of social action: Studies in conversation analysis* (pp. 21–27). Cambridge: Cambridge University Press.

Sacks, H. (1987). On the preference for agreement and contiguity in sequences in conversation. In G. Button & J. R. E. Lee (Eds.), *Talk and social organization* (pp. 54–85). Clevedon, England: Multilingual Matters.

Sacks, H., Schegloff, E. A., & Jefferson, G. (1974). A simplest systematics for the organization of turn-taking for conversation. *Language, 50,* 696–735.

Satariano, W. A, Ragheb, N. E., & Dupuis, M. H. (1989). Comorbidity in older women with breast cancer: An epidemiologic approach. In R. Yancik & J. W. Yates (Eds.), *Cancer in the elderly: Approaches to early detection and treatment* (pp. 71–107). New York: Springer.

Schegloff, E. A. (1972). Notes on conversational practice: Formulating place. In D. Sudnow (Ed.), *Studies in social interaction* (pp. 75–119). New York: Free Press.

Schegloff, E. A. (1982). Discourse as an interactional achievement: Some uses of "uh huh" and other things that come between sentences. In D. Tannen (Ed.), *Analyzing discourse: Text and talk.* Georgetown University Roundtable on Languages and Linguistics (pp. 71–93). Washington, DC: Georgetown University Press.

Schegloff, E. A. (1987). Recycled turn beginnings: A precise repair mechanism in conversation's turn-taking organization. In G. Button & J. R. E. Lee (Eds.), *Talk and social organization* (pp. 75–85). Clevedon, England: Multilingual Matters.

Schegloff, E. A. (1992). On talk and its institutional occasions. In P. Drew & J. Heritage (Ed.), *Talk at work: Interactions in institutional settings* (pp. 101–134). Cambridge: Cambridge University Press.

Schegloff, E. A. (1993). Reflections on quantification in the study of conversation. *Research on Language and Social Interaction, 26*(1), 99–128.

Schegloff, E. A. (1997). Whose text? Whose context? *Discourse and Society.* 8(2), 165–187.

Schegloff, E. A., & Sacks, H. (1973). Opening up closings. *Semiotica, 8*(4), 289–327.

Schiffrin, D. (1987). *Discourse markers.* Cambridge: Cambridge University Press.

Silliman, R. A., Balducci, L., Goodwin, J. S., Holmes, F. F., & Leventhal, E. A. (1993). Breast cancer care in old age: What we know, don't know, and do. *Journal of the National Cancer Institute, 85*(3), 190–199.

Silliman, R. A., Guadagnoli, A. E., & Weitberg, A. B., & Mor, V. (1989). Age as a predictor of diagnostic and initial treatment intensity in newly diagnosed breast cancer patients. *Journal of Gerontology, 44,* M46–M50.

Silverman, D., Bor, R., Miller, R., & Goldman, E. (1991). "Obviously the advice is then to keep to safer sex": Advice-giving and advice reception in AIDS counselling. In P. Aggleton, P. Davies, & G. Hart (Eds.), *AIDS: Rights, risk, and reason* (pp. 174–191). Bristol, PA: Taylor & Francis, Falmer Press.

Siminoff, L. A. (1987). Description and correlates of breast cancer adjuvant treatment decisions. Unpublished Ph.D. dissertation, Johns Hopkins University, Baltimore.

Siminoff, L. A., & Fetting, J. H. (1989). Effects of outcome framing on treatment decisions in the real world. *Medical Decision Making, 9,* 262–271.

Siminoff, L. A., & Fetting, J. H. (1991). Factors affecting treatment decisions for a life-threatening illness: The case of medical treatment of breast cancer. *Social Science and Medicine, 32*(7), 813–818.

Siminoff, L. A., Fetting, J. H., & Abeloff, M. D. (1989). Doctor-patient communication about breast cancer adjuvant therapy. *Journal of Clinical Oncology 7*(9), 1192–1200.

Skipper, J. K. (1965). Communication and the hospitalized patient. In J. K. Skipper & R. C. Leonard (Eds.), *Social interaction and patient care* (pp. 61–82). Philadelphia: Lippincott.

Smith, C. K., Polis, E., & Hadac, R. R. (1981). Characteristics of the initial medical interview associated with patient satisfaction and understanding. *Journal of Family Practice, 12*(2), 283–288.

Steele, D. J., Jackson, T. C., & Guntmann, M. C. (1990). Have you been taking your pills? The adherence monitoring sequence in the medical interview. *Journal of Family Practice, 30*, 294–299.

Svarstad, B. L. (1979). Physician-patient communication and patient conformity with medical advice. In G. L. Albrecht & P. C. Higgins (Eds.), *Health, illness, and medicine: A reader in medical sociology* (pp. 243–259). Boston: Houghton- Mifflin.

Tannen, D., & Wallat, C. (1983). Doctor/mother/child communication: Linguistic analysis of a pediatric interaction. In S. Fisher & A. Dundas Todd (Eds.), *The social organization of doctor-patient communication* (pp. 203–219). Washington, DC: Center for Applied Linguistics.

ten Have, P. (1991). Talk and institution: A reconsideration of the "asymmetry" of doctor-patient interaction. In D. H. Zimmerman & D. Boden (Eds.), *Talk and social structure: Studies in ethnomethodology and conversation analysis* (pp. 138–163). Cambridge: Polity Press.

Todd, A. D. (1984). The prescription of contraception: Negotiations between doctors and patients. *Discourse Processes, 7*, 171–200.

Trostle, J. A. (1988). Medical compliance as an ideology. *Social Science and Medicine, 27*(12), 1299–1308.

Verhoef, M. J., & Casebeer, A. L. (1997). Broadening horizons: Integrating quantitative and qualitative research. *Canadian Journal of Infectious Disease, 8*(2), 65–66.

West, C. (1983). "Ask me no questions . . ." An analysis of queries and replies in physician-patient dialogues. In S. Fisher & A. Todd (Eds.), *The social orga-*

nization of doctor-patient communication (pp. 75–106). Washington, DC: Center for Applied Linguistics.

West, C. (1984a). Medical misfires: Mishearings, misgivings, and misunderstandings in physician-patient dialogues. *Discourse Processes, 7*, 107–134.

West, C. (1984b). *Routine complications: Troubles with talk between doctors and patients*. Bloomington: Indiana University Press.

West, C., & Frankel, R. (1991). Miscommunication in medicine. In N. Coupland, H. Giles, & J. Wiemann (Eds.), *Miscommunication and problematic talk* (pp. 166–194). Newbury Park, CA: Sage.

Yancik, R., Ries, L. G., & Yates, J. W. (1989). Breast cancer in aging women: A population-based study of contrasts in stage, surgery, and survival. *Cancer, 63,* 976–981.

Zimmerman, D. H. (1984). Talk and its occasion: The case of calling the police. In D. Schiffrin (Ed.), *Meaning, form, and use in context: Linguistics applications.* Georgetown University Roundtable on Language and Linguistics (pp. 210–228). Washington, DC: Georgetown University Press.

Zimmerman, D. H. (1992). The interactional organization of calls for emergency assistance. In P. Drew & J. Heritage (Eds.), *Talk at work: Interaction in institutional settings* (pp. 418–469). Cambridge: Cambridge University Press.

Zimmerman, D. H., & Boden, D. (1991). Structure-in-action: An introduction. In D. H. Zimmerman & D. Boden (Eds.), *Talk and social structure: Studies in ethnomethodology and conversation analysis* (pp. 3–21). Cambridge: Polity Press.

Index